Guide to Genital HPV Diseases and Prevention

Guide to
Genital HPV Diseases and Prevention

Edited by
William Bonnez
University of Rochester School of Medicine and Dentistry
Rochester, New York, USA

informa
healthcare

New York   London

Informa Healthcare USA, Inc.
52 Vanderbilt Avenue
New York, NY 10017

© 2009 by Informa Healthcare USA, Inc.
Informa Healthcare is an Informa business

No claim to original U.S. Government works
Printed and bound in India by Replika Press Pvt. Ltd.
10 9 8 7 6 5 4 3 2 1

International Standard Book Number-10: 1-4398-0899-6 (Softcover)
International Standard Book Number-13: 978-1-4398-0899-3 (Softcover)

Library of Congress Cataloging-in-Publication Data

Guide to genital HPV diseases and prevention / edited by William Bonnez.
    p. ; cm.
  Includes bibliographical references.
  ISBN-13: 978-1-4200-9477-0 (softcover: alk. paper)
  ISBN-10: 1-4200-9477-7 (softcover: alk. paper) 1. Papillomavirus diseases.
2. Generative organs—Infections. I.
Bonnez, William.
  [DNLM: 1. Genital Neoplasms, Female—prevention & control. 2.
Papillomavirus Infections—prevention & control. 3. Genital Neoplasms,
Male—prevention & control. 4. Papillomaviridae—pathogenicity. WP 145
G946 2008]
  RC168.P15G85 2008
  614.5'81–dc22

                            2008045996

For Corporate Sales and Reprint Permissions call 212-520-2700 or write to: Sales Department, 52 Vanderbilt Avenue, 16th floor, New York, NY 10017.

Visit the Informa Web site at
www.informa.com

and the Informa Healthcare Web site at
www.informahealthcare.com

Dedication

To four of my most cherished guides:

Antoine Bertran who, generous and selfless, opened wide my adolescent mind.

Marthe Vigneau, my grandmother, whose example of hard labor and love resonates with her death as this book goes to press.

My mother, Jeanne, an eternal cheery and loving supporter. My late father, Jean, for his moral courage and generosity.

Preface

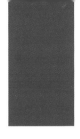

Fifty years ago, the statement "a wart is a wart" would have been to many physicians an apt summary of all there was to know about human papillomavirus (HPV). Cutaneous and genital warts have been known since Antiquity. Their transmissible nature was demonstrated in 1895. In 1907, the agent was shown to be a virus whose first electron micrographs were obtained in 1942. Research progressed in the 1930s and 1940s, but it was with animal papillomaviruses. This is when the link between the cottontail rabbit papillomavirus (Shope papillomavirus) and cancer was established.

Unfortunately, for the following 30 years the consensus became that humans were different and that no viruses played a role in their cancers. This perception began to change in the 1970s. It was first noted that epidermodysplasia verruciformis, a rare genodermatosis whose lesions are caused by HPV and often transform into squamous cell carcinomas, could be a model of HPV oncogenesis. A similar causal association was then conjectured between HPV and cervical cancer. Harald zur Hausen was awarded the 2008 Nobel Prize of Medicine and Physiology for this insight. At the time herpes simplex virus was thought to be the best culprit.

Between 1977 and 1985, a series of observations established that more than one type of HPV existed, and each had a particular disease association. For example, HPV-6 and -11 were isolated from external genital warts, and their DNAs were cloned and sequenced. Nevertheless, it was the isolation of HPV-16 and -18 in cervical cancer lesions that provided the first clear evidence for a causal link between these viruses and genital cancer.

The basic principles of papillomavirus molecular and cellular oncogenesis were quickly established by the beginning of the 1990s. That decade saw the rapid development of the many epidemiologic studies that solidified and complemented the proofs that some genital (also called mucosal) HPV caused cervical cancer. With more limited, but mounting evidence, other cancers were also added to the list, such as cancers of the vulva, vagina, penis, anus, and more recently of the oropharynx.

By the late 1990s, preclinical and early clinical studies indicated that a preventive vaccine could be developed. The first evidence of the clinical efficacity of this vaccine to prevent HPV-16 cervical infections was presented in 2004, and the results were spectacular. The vaccine provided complete protection. Since 2006, two HPV vaccines have come on to the market worldwide after showing virtually complete protection against the precursor lesions of cervical cancer caused by HPV-16 or -18, and, for one of these two vaccines, against external genital warts caused by HPV-6 or -11.

In 30 years of research, knowledge has flourished, and progress has been tangible and remarkable. A wart is no longer just a wart. Only five years ago, health care providers could be ignorant about HPV and still provide proper care. This is not the case any longer, and patients know it. The purpose of this guide is to offer health care providers a readable and accessible source of information on genital HPVs to answer their patients' questions, and help them manage the infections and diseases caused by these viruses. Some emphasis has been placed on HPV immunization, because it is largely the availability of the new vaccines that has rendered this information necessary. In order to produce this book and guarantee the proper expertise, we have assembled a group of physicians and scientists who have all been engaged in HPV research. However, this is not a book for the specialist. Our audience is the novice and interested clinicians, who in the fields of general practice, family medicine, pediatrics, adolescent medicine, obstetrics, gynecology, internal medicine, dermatology, oncology, or urology for instance, are confronted with genital HPV. We wish to hear and learn from these readers if we have attained our goals, and to know how to improve this work.

William Bonnez, M.D.

Contents

Contributors

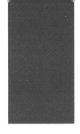

Darron R. Brown

Department of Microbiology and Immunology, Indiana University School of Medicine, Indianapolis, Indiana, U.S.A.

William Bonnez

Infectious Diseases Division, Department of Medicine, University of Rochester School of Medicine and Dentistry, Rochester, New York, U.S.A.

Patti E. Gravitt

Departments of Epidemiology and Molecular Microbiology and Immunology, Johns Hopkins Bloomberg School of Public Health, Baltimore, Maryland, U.S.A.

Cynthia M. Rand

Division of General Pediatrics, Department of Pediatrics, University of Rochester School of Medicine and Dentistry, Rochester, New York, U.S.A.

Robert C. Rose

Infectious Diseases Division, Departments of Medicine, and Microbiology and Immunology, University of Rochester School of Medicine and Dentistry, Rochester, New York, U.S.A.

Mark H. Stoler

Division of Surgical Pathology, Department of Pathology, University of Virginia Health System, Charlottesville, Virginia, U.S.A.

Eugene P. Toy

Gynecologic Oncology, Department of Obstetrics and Gynecology, University of Rochester School of Medicine and Dentistry, Rochester, New York, U.S.A.

Introduction

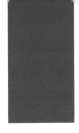

HPV are DNA viruses that infect the stratified squamous epithelia of man. More than 100 genotypes have been fully characterized and the list is growing. It is now clear that these infections are extremely common, perhaps universal, but also mostly exist at a low, latent level causing no detectable alterations to the tissues. HPVs are distributed throughout the body (Figure 1), but with different anatomic predilections that allow to distinguish three major groups of HPV-associated diseases and viruses: (1) the HPV types found in cutaneous warts, such as plantar, common, and flat warts; (2) those associated with epidermodysplasia verruciformis, a rare genodermatosis; and (3) the HPVs associated with genital or mucosal lesions. This guide is devoted to this third group of conditions that includes genital warts, laryngeal papillomas, as well as precancers (also called dysplasias or intraepithelial neoplasias) and cancers of the uterine cervix, vagina, vulva, penis, anus, and of the head and neck area. Among the almost 40 genital HPV genotypes, types 6 and 11 are predominantly responsible for the benign diseases, and types 16 and 18 for the malignancies. Genital HPV infections cause a significant health burden, if only because cervical cancer is the second most common and lethal cancer detected in women worldwide.

Chapter 1 describes the virology of HPV and the basic mechanisms by which it can elude the immune system and cause cancer. Patient counseling draws largely on the knowledge of descriptive epidemiology, transmission, and natural history, topics addressed in chapter 2. The HPV-associated diseases are described in chapter 3, with an emphasis on the most common ones. Treatment of these lesions, when appropriate, is still largely based on various destructive or excisional methods, none of them entirely satisfactory, as discussed in chapter 4.

The diagnosis of external lesions is mostly clinical, but for internal lesions or in situations involving immunocompromised patients [e.g., those infected with the human immunodeficiency virus (HIV), or the recipients of allogeneic grafts] adjunctive diagnostic tools are used (chap. 5). These diagnostics tools are also used in screening for cancer. Cervical cytology was disseminated into common practice after 1947 in the United States,

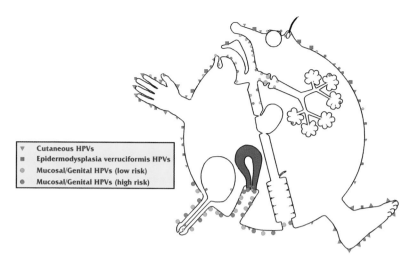

Figure 1 Anatomic distribution of the different human papillomaviruses.

owing to George Papanicolaou's efforts. The Pap smear, as it is also known, is still the key tool for the prevention of cervical cancer. However, screening has become complex (chap. 6), and HPV DNA testing is now part of it. Screening is also gaining ground in the prevention of anal cancer in the HIV-infected population.

Preventing HPV infection before it reaches the disease stage remains the ideal. There is now very clear evidence of the modest but clinically significant effectiveness of the male condom in preventing genital HPV infections and diseases. However, the most significant development in the HPV field has been the availability of very effective vaccines since June 2006 (chap. 7). Two vaccines are now available in many countries, both based on the concept of virus-like particles (VLPs). One, Gardasil, is directed at HPV types 6 and 11, which account for 80% of external genital warts, and at HPV-16 and -18, responsible for 70% of cervical cancer. The other vaccine, Cervarix, is directed at only HPV-16 and -18. Because HPV is a necessary cause of cervical cancer, these vaccines, and future, more polyvalent formulations, hold the promise of quasi-eradication of this cancer. This would change and possibly eliminate screening. But all the other cancers attributed to the same oncogenic HPV types, and for which screening does not exist, are also likely to disappear, especially if both males and females are immunized. Gathering the evidence supporting these expectations is the challenge of the coming years. The other challenge is economic, and is to make these presently costly vaccines available to the countries that often need them the most. The experience with the hepatitis B vaccine is encouraging, because costs have dropped.

In preparing this publication my gratitude goes to the authors for accepting tight deadlines and imperious decisions, and to the staff at Informa, Maria Lorusso, Daniel Falatko, Sandra Beberman, and Brian Kearns for their patience and advice.

William Bonnez, M.D.

Biology

Robert C. Rose
Infectious Diseases Division, Departments of
Medicine, and Microbiology and Immunology,
University of Rochester School of Medicine and
Dentistry, Rochester, New York, U.S.A.

Mark H. Stoler
Division of Surgical Pathology, Department of
Pathology, University of Virginia Health System,
Charlottesville, Virginia, U.S.A.

1.1. Virology

1.1.1. Basic Virology

Papillomaviruses are small, round, non-enveloped DNA viruses that infect mammals, birds and reptiles, with species- and tissue-specificity. They are one of the oldest, largest, and most diverse of the known virus families. Human papillomaviruses (HPVs), like all papillomaviruses, target the stratified squamous epithelia of the body. A subset is also able to infect the glandular epithelium of the cervix.

1.1.1.1. Structure

The virion consists of a single molecule of circular, double-stranded DNA about 8 kilobasepairs in length, contained within a symmetric icosahedral protein coat, the capsid, which is made by the spontaneous assembly of the L1 major and L2 minor capsid proteins (Fig. 1.1).

1.1.1.2. Classification and Disease Association

Papillomaviruses belongs to the *Papillomaviridae* family. Because culture of these viruses is not readily available, taxonomy is based on genotyping and not serotyping, which is traditionally used in virology. Genotypes are considered distinct if they share less than 90% homology in the DNA sequence of the open reading frame (ORF), coding for the major capsid protein. Subtypes have between 90% and 95% homology, and variants between 96% and 98%. The *Papillomaviridae* family has 18 genera. The human papillomaviruses belong to the *Alpha-*, *Beta-*, *Gamma-*, *Mu-*, and *Nupapillomavirus*. They are numbered in order of discovery.

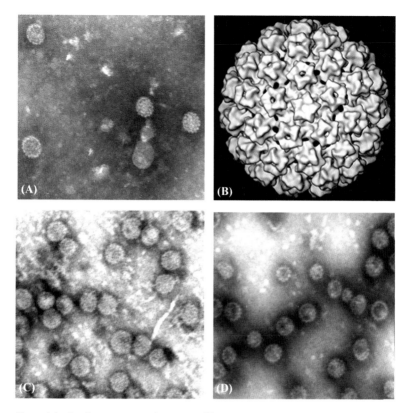

Figure 1.1 *Papillomavirus capsid structure. (**A**) Electron micrograph of native HPV11 virions (Courtesy W. Bonnez); (**B**) cryoelectron micrograph of a BPV1 virion; (**C**) electron micrographs of HPV16; and (**D**) HPV18 L1 virus-like particles (VLPs). Source: For parts A, B: http://commons.wikimedia.org/wiki/Image:Papillomavirus_capsid.png. For parts C, D: Source: Rose RC, Bonnez W, Da Rin C, McCance DJ, Reichman RC. Serological differentiation of human papillomavirus types 11, 16 and 18 using recombinant virus-like particles. J Gen Virol 1994; 75:2445–2449.*

At least 111 HPV have been officially recognized, but this is rapidly changing, and the actual number is thought to be considerably higher. Although different HPVs infect different anatomic sites and have different disease-associations (Table 1.1), many of the most recently identified HPV genotypes do not have a clear pathogenic role, and do not appear in Table 1.1. Although not completely reflective of phylogeny, it is convenient to classify HPVs into three groups according to associated diseases. Members of the first group of HPVs are responsible for the very common

Table 1.1 HPV Types and Disease Associations

Disease	Frequent association	Less frequent association
Cutaneous warts	1, 2, 4	3, 7, 10, 26, 27, 28, 29, 38, **41**[a], 49, 57, 63, 65, 75, 76, 77,80, 83, 84, 86, 87
Epidermodysplasia verruciformis	**5, 8**, 9, 12, **14**, 15, **17**	19, **20**, 21–25, 36–38, **47**, 49, 50, 93
Condylomata acuminata	6, 11	**30**, 42, 43, 44, **45**, **51**, 54, 55, 70
Intraepithelial neoplasias	6, 11, **16**, **18**	**30**, **31**, **33**, 34, **35**, **39**, 40, 42, 43, 44, **45**, **51–53**, **56**, 57, **58**, **59**, 61, 62, 64, **66**, 67, **68**, 69, 71, 72, 74, **82**
Carcinomas	**16**, **18**	**31**, **33**, **35**, **39**, **45**, **51**, **52**, **56**, **58**, **59**, **66**, **67**, **68**, **70**, **73**, **82**

[a]The genotypes in bold have an established or possible oncogenic potential.

cutaneous warts (hand, plantar, and flat warts). These viruses are found only rarely in the genital tract. Members of the second group are found in a rare genodermatosis, epidermodysplasia verruciformis, whereby associated lesions have a high propensity in adulthood to develop into squamous cell cancers in the sun-exposed areas of the body. These viruses are also frequently present in the normal skin.

The third group is made of the genital HPVs, also called mucosal HPVs, because they infect the mucous membranes of not only the anogenital tract, but also of the upper aerodigestive tract. The genital papillomaviruses belong to the *Alphapapillomavirus* genus. Their phylogeny is shown in Figure 1.2. Within the genus, different species are recognized, each with a representative genotype. For the purpose of this book, it is important to recognize that HPV-6 is the representative type of species 10, to which HPV-11 also belongs; HPV-16 is the representative of species 9, and HPV-18 of species 7. What accounts for tissue tropism is not well understood.

1.1.1.3. Papillomavirus Genomic Organization
Viral open reading frames are arrayed in a linear fashion on only one strand of the double-stranded circular DNA genome (Fig. 1.3). Viral genome functioning is controlled by the so-called "upstream regulatory region" (URR), which contains many binding sequences for cellular and viral

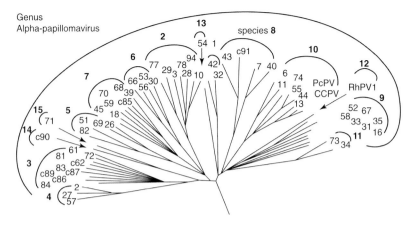

Figure 1.2 Phylogeny of the Alphapapillomavirus genus. Source: *From de Villiers EM, Fauquet C, Broker TR, Bernard HU, zur Hausen H. Classification of papillomaviruses. Virology 2004; 324:17–27.*

factors that alone or in concert orchestrate the selective synthesis of viral messages and the replication of the viral genome. Genomic organization is well conserved among all HPVs, with Early ("E") and Late ("L") ORF regions that are capable of coding viral proteins, following the URR.

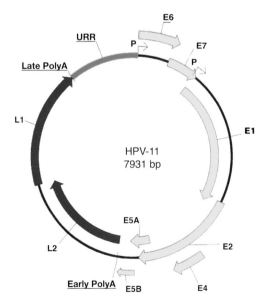

Figure 1.3 Genomic organization of a representative papillomavirus genotype (HPV-11).

Table 1.2 HPV Viral Proteins Main Functions

	Protein[a]	Function(s)
"Early" proteins	E1	Viral DNA replication Maintenance of episomal state Control of gene transcription
	E2	Control of viral transcription and DNA replication Inhibition of E6 and E7, and activation of E2 N-terminus gene expression
	E4	Not well defined, but interact with the cellular intermediate filaments
	E5	Enhances growth factor effects Immune evasion
	E6[b]	Destroys p53, a tumor suppressor protein that represses the cell cycle Inhibits apoptosis Contributes to immune evasion
	E7[b]	Inactivates the retinoblastoma protein, a tumor suppressor protein that represses the cell cycle Contributes to immune evasion
"Late" proteins	L1	Major capsid structural protein, pentamer/capsid self-assembly
	L2	Minor capsid structural protein (virion assembly and infectivity)

[a]There is no E3 protein.
[b]The interaction of E6 and E7 with tumor suppressor proteins is limited to high-risk HPVs.

(Fig. 1.3). The names Early and Late refers loosely to when the messages and proteins from these ORFs appear during viral infection.

1.1.1.4. Viral Proteins

Viral ORFs in both the E and L regions are named according to decreasing size. Thus, E1 and L1 are the largest of the E and L region viral proteins, respectively. The main known and suspected functional properties of the various viral proteins are listed in Table 1.2.

1.1.1.5. Growth in Cell Culture and Animal Model Systems

Due to strict species- and tissue-specificities of these viruses and their requirement for differentiating epithelium for completion of the viral life cycle, growth of HPV genotypes in the laboratory for a long time was impossible, and remains difficult and complex. This is why for research purposes, one still relies on animal papillomavirus models such as the cottontail rabbit papillomavirus, the bovine papillomavirus, and the canine oral papillomavirus. HPV-1, then HPV-11, and later HPV-16 were first grown, beginning in 1985, by infecting small fragments of human epithelial tissue (mostly neonatal foreskin), and implanting them under the renal capsule of immunodeficient mice (athymic "nude" mice or animals with the severe combined immunodeficiency syndrome). In this type of model the viral infection recapitulates the macroscopic, microscopic, and molecular features of a natural infection. It has been possible since, to grow HPV in skin organotypic (artificial skin) culture systems.

1.1.1.6. Antigenicity

All HPV proteins are immunogenic and thus capable of eliciting both humoral and cellular immune responses. In natural infection, tight regulatory control over viral gene expression acts to minimize antigen exposure in the infected host; thus, the magnitude of such responses usually is quite low. Although both the E6 and E7 proteins of the high-risk HPVs are continually expressed in neoplastic lesions, E6-specific cellular responses are more often associated with disease resolution than are similar responses against the viral E7 protein. The L1 major capsid protein displays a common (shared across all papillomaviruses tested) linear epitope when denatured that usually is not seen by the immune system in natural infection. By contrast, the L1 protein in its native conformation is immunogenic. It can readily assemble into an empty capsid in the absence of L2, the minor capsid protein. This empty capsid when made in vitro is called a virus-like particle (VLP) and is the basis of the current vaccine (Fig. 1.1). These VLPs have the same immunologic properties as the infectious virions. They possess immunodominant antigenic sites that generate a strong binding and neutralizing antibody response that is generally genotype-specific. The second structural and functional component of the viral capsid, the L2 minor capsid protein, also possesses neutralizing epitopes within the amino-terminal region. These epitopes are linear, much less immunogenic, but broadly cross-reactive among alternate virus genotypes.

1.2. Pathogenesis

1.2.1. Molecular and Cellular Pathogenesis

The hallmark of a symptomatic HPV infection is to produce a proliferation of the stratified squamous epithelium. This proliferation might be benign, but a subgroup of HPV types (Table 1.1) can also cause a malignant tissue proliferation. They are called high-risk HPVs. This malignant process, which ultimately results in a squamous cell carcinoma, but also in the case

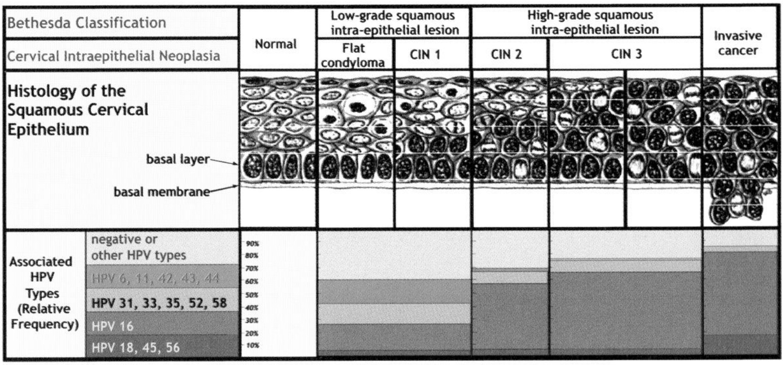

Bethesda Classification			Low-grade squamous intra-epithelial lesion		High-grade squamous intra-epithelial lesion		Invasive cancer
Cervical Intraepithelial Neoplasia		Normal	Flat condyloma	CIN 1	CIN 2	CIN 3	
Histology of the Squamous Cervical Epithelium basal layer basal membrane							
Associated HPV Types (Relative Frequency)	negative or other HPV types	90%					
	HPV 6, 11, 42, 43, 44	80% 70% 60%					
	HPV 31, 33, 35, 52, 58	50% 40%					
	HPV 16	30% 20%					
	HPV 18, 45, 56	10%					

Figure 1.4 *The relationship between terminology histology and various HPV types.* Source: *Modified from Bonnez W. Papillomavirus. In: Richman RD, et al., eds. Clinical Virology. 2nd ed. Washington, DC: American Society for Microbiology; 2002:557–596.*

of the cervix in an adenocarcinoma, starts with precursor lesions. These precursor lesions were originally called *dysplasias*, but now the term of intraepithelial neoplasia is favored. The differences between the two nomenclatures are detailed in chapter 5 (see Table 5.2).

Three grades of intraepithelial neoplasia are recognized from the less severe, grade 1, to the most severe, grade 3. Although it may have seemed originally that the progression from grade 1 to grade 3 and eventually to cancer is linear and progressive, this is not necessarily so. In the case of the cervix, in recognition of the lessons learned in the past couple of decades, it appears more meaningful for screening and management purposes to distinguish cervical intraepithelial neoplasia grade 1 (CIN1) from CIN2 and CIN3. This change was incorporated in the Bethesda system (see chap. 5, Fig. 1.4). Underlying this difference are the mix of HPV genotypes present in these lesions. In CIN1 two-thirds of the HPV types are high-risk, but one third is low-risk. In CIN2 and particularly CIN3, the vast majority of HPV types are high risk. In invasive cervical cancer they are all high-risk by definition, but among these high-risk types HPV-16 and -18 becomes much more predominant, accounting for 70% of the cases. This clearly shows that even among high-risk HPVs some are more oncogenic than other. The most oncogenic, HPV-16, is about 460-fold more likely to be present in a cancerous cervix than in a nomal cervix. In comparison, tobacco smoking increases the risk of lung cancer by only 20-fold.

Not only is HPV DNA present in every pathology linked to HPV, but also most importantly, HPV messenger RNA is expressed in these lesions. The presence of viral RNA and protein expression and the interaction of viral proteins with cellular processes leads to a rational framework of viral pathogenesis. Patterns of viral mRNA expression vary with morphology in a tightly regulated and differentiation dependent manner. In low-grade lesions, all viral genes are expressed as a manifestation of vegetative viral replication. In contrast, in HSIL and invasive cancer, there is a restricted pattern of viral gene expression such that E6 and E7 predominate.

Active transcription of HPV DNA within lesions establishes a strong molecular association of HPV with cervical neoplasia. Furthermore, high-risk HPV types are more capable of transforming epithelial cell lines. The essential part of the viral genome for these effects is the expression of the E6 and/or E7 region which as noted in prior sections are more "potent" in their inactivation of the regulatory proteins p53 and pRb respectively compared to low-risk viruses. There is also a strong association between the physical state of HPV DNA within the cell nucleus and the malignant potential of the associated epithelial proliferation. In low-grade lesions, the viral DNAs exist as extrachromosomal plasmids, mostly as monomeric circular molecules. However, in most cancers, HPV DNAs are integrated into host chromosomes. Viral integration most frequently disrupts the E2 ORF, which encodes the transcription regulatory proteins. Loss of these regulatory proteins is thought to be the basis for potential dysregulation of the expression of the transforming E6 and E7 ORFs (Fig. 1.5). This

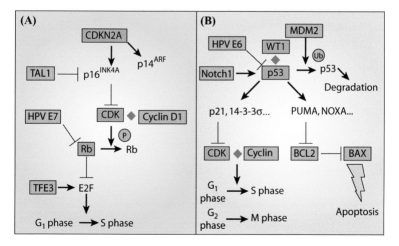

Figure 1.5 The HPV oncogenes E6 and E7 target the inactivation of p53 and pRb respectively These interactions in cells that can still divide leads to the induction of the proliferative phenotype characteristic of cervical precancer. Source: From Figure 2 in Vogelstein B, Kinzler KW. Cancer genes and the pathways they control. Nat Med 2004; 10(8):789–799.

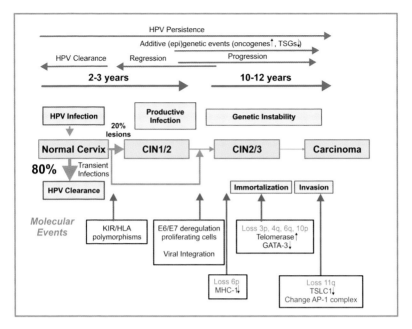

Figure 1.6 *Progression model of cervical cancer based on in vitro transformation steps and data from clinical samples. See text for further description. Potential relevant genetic alterations are indicated in red.* Abbreviations: *TSGs, tumor suppressor genes; HLA, human leukocyte antigen; MHC, major histocompatibility complex; KIR, GATA-3, and TSLC1 are genes likely affected by HPV infection, ↑, indicates increased activity resulting from (epi)genetic alteration(s); ↓, indicates decreased activity resulting from (epi)genetic alteration (s), such as deletion or promoter hypermethylation.* Source: *Modified from Figure 5 in Snijders et al. (2006).*

knowledge permits to build a molecular model for HPV induced carcinogenesis that relates the interaction of HPV gene products with the tightly regulated network of cellular genes involved in the control of cell proliferation (Fig. 1.6).

1.2.1.1. Active Infection

Active HPV infection begins with infection of the "basal or stem" cell population of the cervical transformation zone, cells with the potential to differentiate along squamous, glandular, or neuroendocrine lines that are responsible for epithelial maintenance. In cells committed to squamous differentiation there is an orderly program of maturation throughout the epithelial thickness both at the morphologic as well as molecular level. The

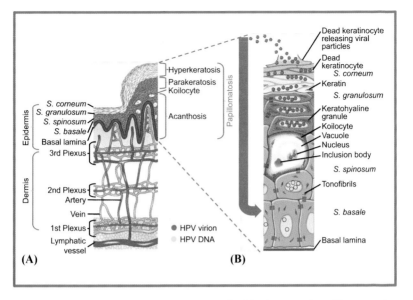

Figure 1.7 Diagram demonstrating the pattern of HPV infection and amplification with squamous epithelial maturation in cutaneous skin. In mucosal sites like the cervix, the stratum corneum is normally absent and the granulosum is less developed but the patterns are otherwise similar. Source: Bonnez W, Reichman RC. Papillomaviruses. In: Mandell GL, et al., eds. Principles and Practice of Infectious Diseases. 6th ed. Philadelphia, PA: Elsevier/Churchill Livingstone, 2005:1841–1856.

only cells capable of cell division in a squamous epithelium are the basal or parabasal cells.

In HPV-infected basal cells, papillomavirus gene expression is inhibited to near maintenance levels and the cells appear nearly normal. Productive HPV gene expression is tightly regulated and permitted only in cells that have begun squamous maturation, with a concomitant loss of proliferative capacity.

In the immediate suprabasal zone there is expression of the early regions of the viral genome, and as the cells differentiate, there is an induction of all viral genes as well as viral DNA synthesis, leading to assembly and production of virions in the cells just beneath the surface (Fig. 1.7).

In the cervix one recognizes such lesions as a low-grade squamous intra-epithelial lesions (LSIL), the biologic equivalent of what has been called mild squamous dysplasia or CIN 1. Koilocytotic atypia in the subsurface cells is a morphologic hallmark of many, but not all of these lesions. Such

LSILs usually regress in a year or so, but rarely persist for extended periods. The nuclear enlargement and hyperchromasia recognized as atypia by pathologists, is a direct result of E6/E7-mediated activation of host DNA synthesis. In a low-grade lesion this is regulated to occur in cells that can no longer divide (i.e., the intermediate squamous cells) and is primarily directed at the production of viral DNA. However, given the small size of the viral genome, even the thousands of copies of the virus present in a productively infected cell cannot account for the two- to fourfold nuclear enlargement that is observed.

It is diagnostically fortunate that ineffective (in the sense of cell division) E6/E7 mediated host DNA synthesis produces the enlarged nuclei and increased nuclear: cytoplasmic (N: C) ratio that one recognizes as abnormal. If the process is not fully developed or is perhaps regressing, then the cells derived from the surface often have less nuclear abnormality (atypical squamous cells of uncertain significance, or ASC-US) than those seen in classical dysplasia. If the cells also have the correct amount and form of the cytokeratin binding protein HPV E4 expressed, then they appear as koilocytes. In the fully developed case, cells with well-developed koilocytotic atypia are classified as being derived from a mild dysplasia/LSIL.

1.2.1.2. Oncogenesis

Given that viral gene expression is so tightly regulated, how do high-grade lesions develop? The morphologic hallmark of high-grade dysplasia/HSIL/CIN2-3 is evidence of abnormal basal-like cell proliferation. In these cells, the coordinate link between differentiation and viral early gene expression is lost. How this occurs is unclear, although it certainly must be a rare event (s) given the relative frequency of low versus high-grade lesions.

When it does occur it is a theoretical dead end for the virus, because HSILs by and large do not make virus. Either viral integration or mutations in HPV E2, such that E2 mediated regulation of E6/E7 expression is lost, causes an uncoupling of viral-cell regulation. The viral oncogenes E6 and E7 are *inappropriately* expressed in a population of cells that retain the capacity to divide, thereby initiating and promoting cell proliferation.

As this population of cells proliferates, it overtakes the epithelium producing lesions that are, by definition, characterized by less orderly squamous maturation and basal-like cell overgrowth with evident mitotic and apoptotic activity. The relative infrequency of these effects is biologically and clinically manifest by the older age of patient with, and the relative rarity of, HSILs versus LSILs. Progression to this proliferative *phenotype* occurs most frequently, albeit not exclusively, with high-risk viral types, and results in the high grade squamous intraepithelial lesions also called moderate squamous dysplasia, severe squamous dysplasia, or squamous carcinoma in situ (CIN 2/3). Thus, the Bethesda System's break between low-grade versus high-grade is a direct extrapolation of the above model. Indeed, from the standpoint of epithelial biology, there is little rationale for separating moderate from severe dysplasia in that the critical break occurs between mild and moderate dysplasia with the switch to a ***proliferative*** as opposed to a differentiated and virally ***productive*** phenotype.

Most of HPVs effects in promoting cancer development seem to occur in the preinvasive stage. In high grade squamous intraepithelial lesions, the proliferating basaloid cells, driven by E6/E7 over expression, are theoretically at much greater risk for the acquisition of additional genetic errors, clonal selection, etc., perhaps under the influence of external mutagens and/or host genetic predisposition, which further promotes the development of the fully malignant phenotype, most often an invasive squamous cell carcinoma (Fig. 1.5). The different subtypes of squamous cancer are probably related to the multi-step and somewhat random nature of the process. The proportion of different types may reflect the relative likelihood of different genetic pathways to a "successful" cancer, in part modulated by the microenvironment in which the lesion develops. Hence, early observations that keratinizing cancers are often more ectocervical than large cell non-keratinizing or small cell malignancies, which tend to originate higher in the endocervical canal, have some contemporary validation.

Given this model for cervical squamous neoplasia, how does one account for the development of other epithelial tumors e.g., glandular and small cell neuroendocrine neoplasms? By analogy, reserve cells that are already committed to glandular differentiation are, because of a lack of an appropriate differentiation environment, not going to be productive of virions. This is apparently because the productive viral life cycle requires the cellular milieu of orderly squamous differentiation. If this is true, then viral infection in cells committed to glandular differentiation most often results (from the viral standpoint) in an abortive or latent infection of morphologically normal endocervical cells, another catastrophe for the virus. Rarely, deregulation of viral early gene expression occurs in these usually nonpermissive cells. This leads to proliferative lesions of glandular cells, which pathologists recognize as severe endocervical dysplasia better known as adenocarcinoma in situ (AIS). There is no biologic correlate in this model of a low-grade glandular dysplasia. Hence, this nicely explains the inability of pathologists to reproducibly recognize, either cytologically or histologically, a clinically meaningful lesion less severe than what most call AIS.

HPV-18 (and perhaps 45 and other related viruses) seems to be more successful at inducing neoplastic proliferation in glandular cells than HPV-16. Perhaps this is because HPV-18 has a greater disposition to integrate into the genome. Or maybe HPV-18 has some receptor-like preference for cells predisposed to other than squamous differentiation. We really do not know. Certainly, no HPV type can be exclusively trophic for non-squamous cells because, under the above model, that virus would be eliminated from the population since virion production requires a squamous milieu.

Again by analogy, depending upon the genetic switches that over time accompany virally induced glandular proliferations, the outcome may be an invasive adenocarcinoma, most often endocervical, but less frequently of another type, e.g., endometrioid or clear cell adenocarcinoma. The relative frequencies of the different types of cervical adenocarcinoma again may just reflect the relative frequency of the different populations committed towards various types of differentiation.

Essentially identical arguments can be made for the development of small cell neuroendocrine carcinomas, tumors that are almost always associated with HPV 18 and whose low incidence probably reflects the relative abundance of a susceptible neuroendocrine-committed precursor cell population and the rarity of "successful" viral induction of cell proliferation in such cells.

1.2.2. Immunology

1.2.2.1. Cellular Innate and Adaptive Response

Many aspects of the cellular immunology of HPV infections are poorly understood. The example of patients with extensive cutaneous verrucosis or with epidermodysplasia verruciformis suggests that several distinct genes probably contribute to the control of genital HPV infections. Among those, some HLA class I (A, B, and Cw), and class II (DB1 and DQB1) haplotypes, or combination thereof, increase (A*0301, B*4402, BB 4402-DRB1*1101-DQB1*0301) or decrease (B*1501, DRB1*1101 and DQB1*0301) the risk of development of cervical squamous cell carcinoma. In addition, there is laboratory evidence that HPV-16 E6 and E7 proteins interact with the toll-like receptor 9, a component of innate immunity.

Langerhans cells which are present in the normal epidermis and are professional antigen-presenting cells are usually decreased in number in HPV lesions. During wart regression there is an increase of the density of Langerhans cells and the presence of a mononuclear cell infiltrate, with lymphocytes displaying activation markers. A chemokine and cytokine response is responsible for stimulating this cellular migration and angiogenesis. The molecules involved include tumor necrosis factor (TNF) alpha, monocyte chemotactic protein 1 (MCP-1), chemokine CCL27, vascular endothelial cell growth factor, interferons alpha, beta, and gamma, interleukins 5 and 8, interferon gamma inducible protein (IP-10), retinoic acid, and tumor growth factor (TGF) beta. Although the trigger for wart regression is unknown, viral proteins E5, E6, and E7 are likely responsible for lesion persistence by interacting directly with some of the chemokines and cytokines listed.

The cellular immune response has specificity as shown by the presence in patients with HPV lesions of a lymphoproliferative response, systemic and local, to the viral proteins, especially E6 and E7. A cytotoxic response can also be detected. These observations have guided the design of therapeutic vaccines (see chap. 4). Natural killer cells are also present in CIN, but the importance of their role is unknown.

1.2.2.2. Humoral Response

The humoral response to HPV infection is better understood. Early viral proteins generate a very weak immune response that is not detected in most patients. However, about half of patients with invasive cervical cancer have antibodies to the E6 and E7 proteins. The strongest immune response during a natural infection is directed to the L1 protein in its native conformation. It is detected in about 50% to 70% of the patients and is a good marker of past or present infection. It is made mostly of IgG, but IgA can also be detected. Some of these antibodies are actually neutralizing, but the levels are generally too low in a natural infection to give a significant immunity to the patient.

Selected References

Snijders PJ, Steenbergen RD, Heideman DA, Meijer CJ. HPV-mediated cervical carcinogenesis: concepts and clinical implications. J Pathol 2006; 208:152–164.
Hebner CM, Laimins LA. Human papillomaviruses: basic mechanisms of pathogenesis and oncogenicity. Rev Med Virol 2006; 16:83–97.
Schiffman M, et al. Human papillomavirus and cervical cancer. Lancet 2007; 370:890–907.
Castle PE, et al. The relationship of community biopsy-diagnosed cervical intraepithelial neoplasia grade 2 to the quality control pathology-reviewed diagnoses: an ALTS report. Am J Clin Pathol 2007; 127:805–815.
Castle PE, et al. Risk assessment to guide the prevention of cervical cancer. Am J Obstet Gynecol 2007; 197:356 e1–e6.

Stoler MH. ASC, TBS, and the power of ALTS. Am J Clin Pathol 2007; 127: 489–491.

Stoler M. The impact of human papillomavirus biology on the clinical practice of cervical pathology. Pathol Case Rev 2005; 10:119–127.

Stoler MH, Schiffman M. Interobserver reproducibility of cervical cytologic and histologic interpretations: realistic estimates from the ASCUS-LSIL Triage Study. JAMA 2001; 285:1500–1505.

Stanley M. Immunobiology of HPV and HPV vaccines. Gynecol Oncol 2008; 109(2 suppl):S15–S21.

Epidemiology

2

Patti E. Gravitt
Departments of Epidemiology and Molecular
Microbiology and Immunology, Johns Hopkins
Bloomberg School of Public Health,
Baltimore, Maryland, U.S.A.

2.1. HPV Disease Burden

Human papillomavirus (HPV) infections are causally associated with a range of human diseases. The alpha-species (also known as mucosal/genital) genotypes broadly infect the epithelium of the anogenital tract and oral cavity of both men and women, including the cervix, vagina, vulva, perineum, anus, penis, and scrotum. The manifestation of HPV infection depends on the site of infection and the HPV genotype (Table 2.1). High-risk HPV types are necessary for the development of cervical and most anal cancers, and are causally related to a subset of oral cancers, especially of the oropharynx. The types defined as high risk continue to evolve with emerging data. In the latest 2007 IARC Monograph on the carcinogenicity of HPV, a consistent association with cancer was found for HPV types 16, 18, 31, 33, 35, 39, 45, 51, 52, 56, 58, 59, and 66, with suggestive evidence of cancer association with HPV types 26, 68, 73, and 82. Figure 2.1 shows the genotype distribution in invasive cervical cancer compared to the subclinical cervical infections in the cytologically normal population. This figure illustrates the relatively higher carcinogenic potential of HPV16, which accounts for more than 50% of cervical cancers and nearly 90% of oral cancers caused by HPV, despite only a modest increase in prevalence in the general population.

In addition to cervical cancer, high-risk HPV infections of the penis, vulva, and vagina can lead to cancer at these sites, though these cancers are very rare. An association between HPV and a now predominant subset of oro-pharyngeal cancers has clearly emerged. Rather than being older and with a history of alcohol and tobacco abuse, these cancer patients are younger and have a history of oral sex and marijuana use. HPV-16 and -18 represent 95% of the types found in these tumors.

Table 2.1 Burden of HPV-Related Disease

Clinical manifestation	Incidence rate[a]	% HPV positive	Predominating causal HPV genotypes
Cervical cancer	8.0[b]	100%	HPV-16 (see Fig. 2.1)
Vulvar cancer	2.1[b]	>50% warty/ basaloid[d] 5% keratinizing	HPV-16
Vaginal cancer	0.6[b]	>50%[d]	HPV-16
Anal cancer	1.7[b]	90%[e]	HPV-16
Penile cancer	0.5[c]	40%[e]	HPV-16
Oral cavity and pharyngeal cancer	10.1[b]	35.6% oropharynx[f] 23.5% larynx 24.0% other oral cavity	HPV-16
Anogenital warts	0.24–13%[d]	100%[d]	HPV-6 and HPV-11
Recurrent respiratory papillomatosis	1.8 adult-onset[d] 4.3 juvenile-onset	100%[d]	HPV-11
Conjunctiva papilloma	unreported	95%[d]	HPV-6 and HPV-11

[a] Per 100,000 except anogenital warts.
[b] US SEER Registry.
[c] Wideroff L, Schottenfeld D. Penile cancer. In: Schottenfeld D, Fraumeni JF, eds. Cancer Epidemiology and Prevention. 3rd ed. Oxford: Oxford University Press, 2006:1068–1074.
[d] IARC (2007).
[e] Parkin and Bray (2006).
[f] Kreimer AR, Clifford GM, Boyle P, Franceschi S. Human papillomavirus types in head and neck squamous cell carcinomas worldwide: a systematic review. Cancer Epidemiol Biomarkers Prev 2005; 14:467–475.

Low-risk HPV infections can produce visible papillomas, or warts, in the anogenital tract, oral cavity, and upper respiratory tract. While posing a significant clinical burden, these infections are rarely life-threatening. The exception is the rare occurrence of recurrent respiratory papillomatosis (RRP); the juvenile onset form of this disease (JORRP) also represents the only form of substantial perinatal transmission of HPV. The incidence of HPV-associated diseases is significantly higher among HIV-positive

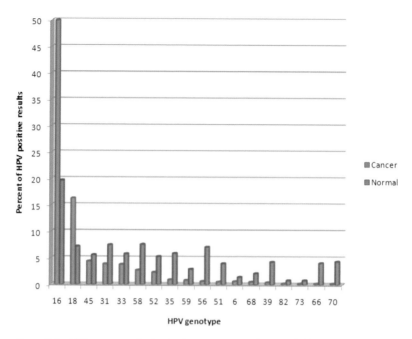

Figure 2.1 HPV genotype distribution in invasive cervical cancer (ICC) versus cytologically negative women, represented as percent of total HPV positive. Source: Clifford et al. 2003, 2005.

individuals, reflecting the importance of T-cell immunity in the control of HPV infections and their manifestations

2.2. HPV Transmission

HPV infects the basal cells of the epithelium. Microtrauma, or microscopic tears to the epithelial barrier, allows access of virus to susceptible cells. In the cervix, this occurs primarily through penetrative sexual intercourse. Non-penetrative genital-to-genital abrasive contact (e.g., heavy petting) may be sufficient for vulvo-vaginal transmission. Consistent condom use offers a relative degree of protection against cervical HPV transmission, however the cumulative incidence associated with consistent condom use is still high (37.8% per year) (see chap. 7). Oral and anal HPV are likely predominately acquired via either direct sexual contact (oral and anal sex) or indirectly by autoinoculation from genital HPV infection. Natural history data suggests that repeat infection between partners is uncommon, probably representing development of some level of natural immunity against re-infection.

2.3. Epidemiology of HPV Infection

Cervical HPV infection has been intensively studied in several well-defined cohorts following the recognition that HPV was a necessary cause of cervical cancer. A causal association between HPV and oral/anal cancers has been more recently established; therefore prospective data on the natural history of oral and anal HPV are limited. The natural history of cervical HPV infection is described below in detail. Since the cross-sectional epidemiology of oral and anal HPV is not identical to cervical HPV caution in extrapolating the cervix data to the natural history of oral and anal HPV is advised.

Estimates of prevalence and incidence of subclinical HPV infection are a function of epithelial sampling, fraction of the sample tested, the sensitivity and genotype spectrum of the HPV assay, and the demographics of the population—contributing to significant variability in the literature. In general, HPV prevalence is highest around the age of sexual debut in women and declines to a nadir in the third decade of life, reflecting the sexual mode of transmission of genital HPV infection and probable development of natural immunity against re-infection (Fig. 2.2). In some countries, a second peak of cervical HPV prevalence is observed beginning in the fourth or fifth decades of life. It is uncertain whether this reflects new sexual exposures or reactivation of latent viral infection acquired at younger ages. A similar age-specific decline in HPV prevalence has not been consistently reported in men, though detection of genital HPV is significantly associated with lifetime and recent sexual partners.

Results from studies of college-aged men and women clearly demonstrate the near ubiquity of HPV infection, the ease of transmission, and the impossibility of defining a particular "at risk" group for HPV infection. The 24-month cumulative incidence for any HPV infection was 38.8% in women and 62.4% in men (Fig. 2.3). Sexual behavior was the strongest risk factor for HPV in both men and women, where HPV incidence increased in men and women reporting more than one sexual partner during follow-up. Importantly, risk associated with a first male partner was similar to that observed by more sexually experienced women; with a cumulative incidence of 50% within three years of contact with a first male sex partner.

Risk of HPV among these "lifetime monogamous" women increased with the male partner's prior sexual experience, highlighting the role of the male partner in risk of female HPV acquisition. These data show that at least 50% of men and women are exposed to HPV within three years of onset of sexual activity, and that even "low risk" monogamous women commonly acquire HPV infection. In studies with longer follow-up and more frequent

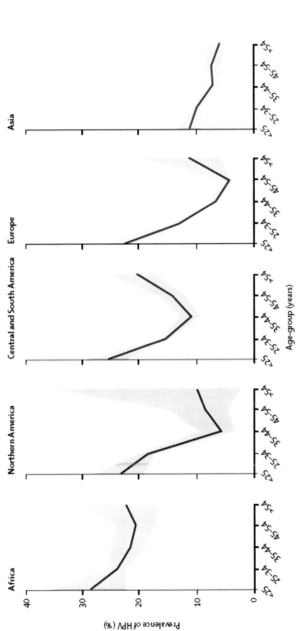

Figure 2.2 Age-specific HPV prevalence by geographic region. Source: de Sanjose S, Diaz M, Castellsague X, et al. Worldwide prevalence and genotype distribution of cervical human papillomavirus DNA in women with normal cytology: a meta-analysis. Lancet Infect Dis 2007; 7:453–459.

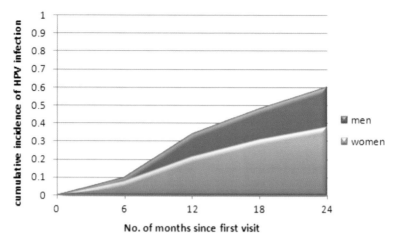

Figure 2.3 Cumulative incidence of genital HPV in college-aged men and women during 24 months of follow-up. Men reported a median of 2 lifetime sexual partners at baseline and women reported a mean of 1.8 sexual partners at baseline. Source: Winer et al. 2003 and Partridge et al. 2007.

sampling, the cumulative HPV exposure is likely to be even higher, with most sexually active adults being exposed to HPV at some point in their lifetimes.

Other factors, including age at sexual debut, cigarette smoking, and use of combined oral contraceptives have been inconsistently associated with an increased risk of HPV acquisition. It is not clear if these factors interact to increase susceptibility of infection given exposure to an infected partner, or if they merely reflect an unmeasured risk of sex with an infected partner.

2.4. Natural History of Cervical HPV Infection

The median duration of a newly detected cervical HPV infection is reported to be approximately 9 to 12 months, with 90% of infections undetectable within 24 months. However, it should be noted that these data are bound by the interval between samples, such that short duration infections (e.g., <3–4 months) would be undetected resulting in overestimation of the median duration of infection. Of more practical use is the estimated duration of prevalent HPV that is identified through cross-sectional screening

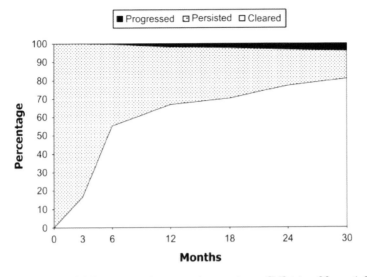

Figure 2.4 HPV clearance, persistence, and progression to CIN2+ in a 30 month follow-up of baseline carcinogenic HPV positive women derived from a population-based cohort in Guanacaste, Costa Rica. Source: Rodriguez AC, Schiffman M, Herrero R, et al. Rapid clearance of human papillomavirus and implications for clinical focus on persistent infections. J Natl Cancer Inst 2008; 100:513–517.

programs. Recent data from an intensively screened, population-based study in Guanacaste, Costa Rica suggest that most prevalent infections also clear rapidly, but that risk of clearance decreases with increasing duration of infection (Fig. 2.4). High-risk HPV infections may have a longer duration compared to low-risk infections, though very long term persistence of low-risk infections is not uncommon. It is not completely clear whether failure to detect HPV infection represents elimination of virus, decline in viral load below the limit of detectability, or development of latent infection. Animal papillomavirus models, however, have been clearly demonstrated to establish lifelong latency in basal epithelial cells which reactivate upon immunosuppression.

Table 2.2 summarizes the absolute risk for progression to CIN 2/3 following a single HPV test result from a younger and older screening population and from a relatively young referral population. These data demonstrate the very low risk of progression in the absence of detectable high-risk HPV within two to three years and the unique risk associated with HPV16 infection. The implications of these data in screening programs are discussed further in chapter 6.

Table 2.2 Absolute Risk Having CIN3 or Cervical Cancer by HPV Status

	Younger women (<30–32 yr) Risk, % (95% CI)		Older women (>30–32 yr) Risk, % (95% CI)	
	Screening population	ASC-US/LSIL referral	Screening population	ASC-US/LSIL referral
HR[a] HPV−	0.2 (0.08–0.3)	1.9 (1.1–3.2)	0.8 (0–0.2)	1.0 (0.4–1.9)
HR HPV+	2.2 (1.3–3.0)	15.9 (14.0–17.8)	4.3 (0–9.9)	12.5 (9.2–16.5)
HR+/ HPV-16−	NA	8.8 (7.1–10.7)	NA	NA
HPV-16+	NA	33.9 (29.2–38.9)	7.2 (4.4–11.0)	36.7 (24.6–50.1)

[a] HR: high risk.

2.5. Natural History of Cervical HPV Infection in HIV-Positive Women

Rates of cervical cancer are significantly increased among women with HIV/AIDS in the United States, according to studies that linked population-based registries for cancer with those for HIV/AIDS. Cross-sectionally, HIV seropositivity is associated with increased prevalence of cervical HPV infection, greater prevalence of precancerous cervical lesions, and with grade of dysplasia. Prospectively, studies have demonstrated that low CD4+ T-cell count and/or high HIV viral load are associated with the incident detection and duration of HPV infection. While sexual exposure remains a significant predictor of HPV infection in the HIV-positive population, new HPV detection rates among women reporting long-term (18 month) abstinence can exceed 20% in the most severely immunosuppressed women, suggesting a proportion of new HPV detected in these women represents reactivation or recrudescence of a previously acquired infection. The increased HPV risk among the HIV-positive women is reflected by a concomitant increase in low-grade cytological abnormalities (CIN1). The incidence of high-grade neoplasia is low even in immunocompromised HIV+ women in long term follow-up with screening, even if significantly greater than in HIV-negatives. While treatment for cervical neoplasia often fails and recurrences are common in women with HIV regardless of the type of treatment, the subsequent lesions are typically low grade. HIV-positive patients should be told not to expect a lasting cure, but that treatment and surveillance result in low risk of cancer.

2.6. Multiple Genotype Infections

It is important to recognize that underlying the estimates of HPV incidence and clearance rates is the fact that concomitant co-infection with several HPV genotypes is common. The prevalence of multiple genotypes among HPV-positive women will vary according the characteristics of the population (age, sexual risk, and HIV prevalence) and with the assays used for genotyping. When methods that detect 37 HPV genotypes are used, 30% to 65% of all HPV positive women are found to be concurrently infected with more than one genotype, highest in young women and women with HIV infection. In a study of women referred with cytologic diagnoses of atypical squamous cells of undetermined significance (ASC-US) or low-grade squamous intraepithelial lesions (LSIL), 56.3% of HPV positive women had multiple type infections. In a population-based sample of 8513 women in Guanacaste, Costa Rica, 31.0% of HPV positive women were co-infected with ≥ 2 concurrent genotypes. In a study of women <25 years seeking health care in Kampala, Uganda, of the HPV positive participants, 38.7% and 64.6% of HIV negative and HIV positive women, respectively, were infected with ≥ 2 HPV genotypes. It is important to keep in mind that these represent prevalent, concurrent infections, and that the cumulative exposure to multiple HPV genotypes over time is likely higher.

2.7. HPV and Cancer—The Causal Link

Attribution of causality to an exposure in complex chronic disease research relies on the cumulative assessment of criteria in several broad areas: the strength and consistency of the association, temporality (i.e., exposure must precede disease onset), and consilience with mechanistic data. The causal link with cervical cancer is now unequivocal. The strength of association as estimated by odds ratios from case-control studies is consistently high, with a summary odds ratio (OR) from a series of case-control studies conducted by the IARC of 83.3. While the OR estimates may vary by study, case-control studies conducted worldwide using validated molecular measurements of HPV exposure are consistent in their support for a strong causal association. The observation that high-risk HPV DNA can be found in nearly 100% of cervical tumor tissues suggests that high-risk HPV is a necessary cause of invasive cervical cancer, a concept which is now well-accepted.

Several large prospective cohort studies have confirmed that HPV exposure precedes the onset of high-grade cervical intraepithelial neoplasia (the most proximate surrogate for invasive cancer that can be ethically measured prior to intervention by lesion excision), clearly establishing the sine qua non of temporality—that exposure precedes disease onset. In vitro demonstration of the interactions of the high-risk viral oncogenes E6 and E7 with several cellular proteins, including inactivation of two critical tumor suppressors (p53 and pRB), reflects the ability of HPV infection to create a cellular environment primed for malignant transformation (see chap. 1). Finally, randomized controlled trials of a prophylactic vaccine against HPV16 and HPV18 have provided rare experimental proof that removal of the putative causal agent prevented nearly 100% of subsequent exposure-associated disease.

2.8. HPV and Cervical Cancer—The Causal Model

Figure 2.5 summarizes the epidemiologic literature into a causal model of cervical cancer. This model reflects the high cumulative exposure to HPV infection and the relatively rare occurrence of CIN up to four to seven years subsequent to HPV detection. From this model, it is clear that additional factors are required to modify host immunologic recognition of high-risk viral infection and progression to a neoplastic phenotype.

Persistent detection of high-risk HPV from exfoliated cervical cells is the strongest risk factor for subsequent high-grade CIN diagnosis. However, persistent HPV detection over a period of years does not appear to predict inevitability of a CIN diagnosis. Epidemiologic study designs are only now

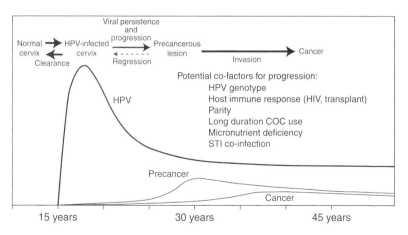

Figure 2.5 *HPV-cervical cancer natural history model and potential co-factors for progression. Source: Modified from Schiffman M, Castle PE. The promise of global cervical-cancer prevention. N Engl J Med 2005; 353:2101–2104.*

beginning to try to distinguish factors affecting risk of HPV persistence from those affecting progression to a neoplastic phenotype.

Previous studies have implicated cigarette smoking, high parity, sexually transmitted infections co-infections (particularly with *Chlamydia trachomatis*), and micronutrient deficiencies as potential factors which interact with high-risk HPV to cause cervical cancer. Of these, cigarette smoking and a history of more than seven full-term births have been consistently found to have an elevated risk for cervical cancer after adjustment for HPV infection. Associations with sexually transmitted co-infections and combined oral contraceptive (COC) use have been inconsistent. Non-causal interpretations of positive associations due to the strong correlation of sexually transmitted infections and COC use with sexual behavior and HPV exposure risk cannot be ruled out for these exposures. However, given the high cumulative exposure to high-risk HPV, it is unlikely that the risk associated with these variables is fully explained by an increased risk in HPV exposure. A recent pooled analysis from the IARC case-control studies confirmed that increased duration of COC use is associated with increased cervical cancer risk, an effect which is attenuated to risk among never users with increasing time since last use. Use of progesterone only contraceptives (e.g., DepoProvera) has not been convincingly associated with an increased risk of invasive cervical cancer. The biological mechanisms attributed to the increased risk associated with these exposures have not been well studied, but the evidence suggests a role of steroid hormones and DNA damaging agents in the etiology of HPV-associated neoplasia.

Selected References
Web Sites

Centers for Disease Control and Prevention. Available at: http://apps.nccd.cdc.gov/ uscs/Table.aspx?Group=TableAll&Year=2004&Display=n.

World Health Organization. Available at: http://www.who.int/hpvcentre. Accessed September 2008.

Articles and Books

IARC. IARC Monographs on the Evaluation of the Carcinogenic Risks to Humans. Lyon: IARC Press, 2007.

Bosch F, Lorincz A, Munoz N, Meijer C, Shah K. The causal relation between human papillomavirus and cervical cancer. J Clin Pathol 2002; 55:244–265.

Clifford GM, Smith JS, Plummer M, Munoz N, Franceschi S. Human papillomavirus types in invasive cervical cancer worldwide: a meta-analysis. Br J Cancer 2003; 88:63–73.

Clifford GM, Gallus S, Herrero R, et al. Worldwide distribution of human papillomavirus types in cytologically normal women in the International Agency for

Research on Cancer HPV prevalence surveys: a pooled analysis. Lancet 2005; 366:991–998.

de Sanjose S, Diaz M, Castellsague X, et al. Worldwide prevalence and genotype distribution of cervical human papillomavirus DNA in women with normal cytology: a meta-analysis. Lancet Infect Dis 2007; 7:453–459.

Gillison ML. Current topics in the epidemiology of oral cavity and oropharyngeal cancers. Head Neck 2007; 29:779–792.

Hernandez BY, McDuffie K, Zhu X, et al. Anal human papillomavirus infection in women and its relationship with cervical infection. Cancer Epidemiol Biomarkers Prev 2005; 14:2550–2556.

Moscicki AB, Schiffman M, Kjaer S, Villa LL. Chapter 5: Updating the natural history of HPV and anogenital cancer. Vaccine 2006; 24(suppl 3):S42–S51.

Munoz N, Bosch F, de Sanjose S, et al. Epidemiologic classification of human papillomavirus types associated with cervical cancer. N Engl J Med 2003; 348:518–527.

Palefsky J, Holly E. Immunosuppression and co-infection with HIV. J Natl Cancer Inst Monogr 2003; 31:41–46.

Parkin DM, Bray F. Chapter 2: The burden of HPV-related cancers. Vaccine 2006; 24(suppl 3):S11–S25.

Partridge JM, Hughes JP, Feng Q, et al. Genital human papillomavirus infection in men: incidence and risk factors in a cohort of university students. J Infect Dis 2007; 196:1128–1136.

Patel P, Hanson DL, Sullivan PS, Novak RM, Moorman AC, Tong TC, et al. Incidence of types of cancer among HIV-infected persons compared with the general population in the United States, 1992–2003. Ann Intern Med 2008; 148:728–736.

Schiffman M, Castle PE, Jeronimo J, Rodriguez AC, Wacholder S. Human papillomavirus and cervical cancer. Lancet 2007; 370:890–907.

Strickler H, Burk R, Fazzari M, et al. Natural history and possible reactivation of human papillomavirus in human immunodeficiency virus-positive women. J Natl Cancer Inst 2005; 97:1–10.

Winer RL, Lee SK, Hughes JP, et al. Genital human papillomavirus infection: incidence and risk factors in a cohort of female university students. Am J Epidemiol 2003; 157: 218–226.

Winer RL, Feng Q, Hughes JP, O'Reilly S, Kiviat NB, Koutsky LA. Risk of female human papillomavirus acquisition associated with first male sex partner. J Infect Dis 2008; 197:279–282.

Diseases

William Bonnez
Infectious Diseases Division, Department of
Medicine, University of Rochester School of
Medicine and Dentistry, Rochester, New York,
U.S.A.

Eugene P. Toy
Gynecologic Oncology, Department of Obstetrics
and Gynecology, University of Rochester School
of Medicine and Dentistry, Rochester, New York,
U.S.A.

3

The clinical manifestations of the mucosogenital HPV infections are the direct consequence of the epithelial proliferation induced by the virus. This proliferation, which is dependent on poorly understood factors, some of which are related to the anatomic location, can protrude to a variable extent above the plane of the normal skin or mucosa, causing papules ranging in height from flat to exuberant. The proliferation also extends below the plane of the epidermis. When limited exclusively to below the tissue surface and benign, it creates an inverted papilloma. Cancers related to HPV can range from fungating to infiltrative, and from small to very large. Therefore, the diagnosis of HPV diseases relies primarily on inspection—sometimes aided by optical magnification and tissue biological stains, and palpation. When lesions are poorly accessible or visible, when malignancy is a concern, or simply when the clinical diagnosis is uncertain, a biopsy is usually the definitive diagnostic tool. For the screening of uterine or anal cancers and the detection of their precursor lesions, the cytology of cells exfoliated from these sites may precede any direct examination and biopsy.

3.1. EXTERNAL ANOGENITAL WARTS

3.1.1. Clinical Manifestations

External genital warts are those HPV-related lesions found in females over the vulva (Fig. 3.1), in the male on the penis (Fig. 3.2) and scrotum, and in both sexes over the mons pubis, the perineum, the anal verge (Fig. 3.3), and the crural folds. They are also designated as venereal warts because of their sexual transmission, but also condylomata acuminata (*singular*, condyloma acuminatum, from the Greek *kondyloma*, meaning knob or knuckle, and

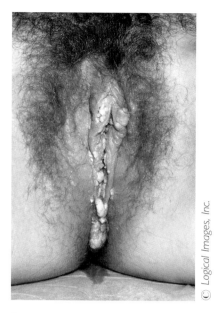

© Logical Images, Inc.

Figure 3.1   *Vulvar condylomata acuminata.*

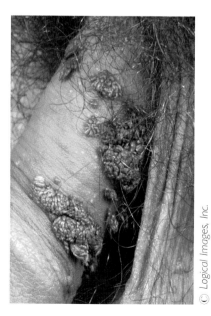

© Logical Images, Inc.

Figure 3.2   *Penile condylomata acuminata.*

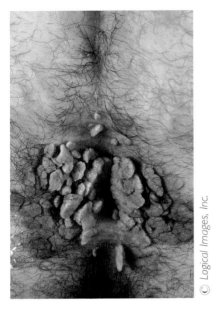

Figure 3.3 Perianal condylomata acuminata.

acuminatum, from the Latin, meaning pointed). The latter term refers to their usual appearance as papillomatous, fleshy lesions with a jagged surface contour. The surface is slightly hyperkeratotic, notably on the keratinized skin, yielding a firm sensation to a glancing touch. The surface contour may be more rounded, mulberry-like. Although the proliferation may on occasion be quite exophytic, forming a spiculated horn, usually the lesion is more likely to be sessile or fungating in appearance, as it might be attached to the skin by a very short peduncle. The lesions can be very flat, better revealed after soaking the tegument with 3% to 5% acetic for one to three minutes (the higher concentration and longer application are reserved for the keratinized skin). While acetowhite macules are not good indicators of HPV-disease, papules that might be overlooked without the application of acetic acid and their whitening are more reliable evidence of an HPV etiology. At diagnosis, individual lesions typically measure from a few millimeters to a couple of centimeters in diameter. They can sometimes reach very large dimensions, exceeding 10 cm in diameter, forming so-called giant condylomas (Fig. 3.4). Most patients present with 3 to 8 lesions, but the total number may sometimes exceed 50, especially in immunodeficient patients. Individual lesions can also coalesce into plaques, leaving hair otherwise absent from single warts to pass through the crevices between lesions. Genital warts have the color of the surrounding tissues with a lighter color for the hyperkeratinized areas. They can also show

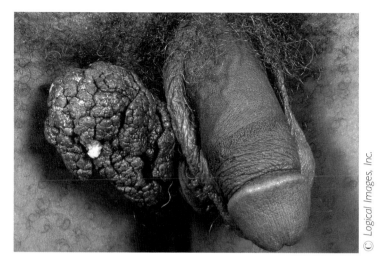

Figure 3.4 Giant condyloma.

various degrees of hyperpigmentation. Frankly pigmented warts deserve particular attention, especially in immunosuppressed or immunodeficient patients as they may in fact be intraepithelial neoplasias associated with oncogenic HPV.

In men warts are mostly found on the penile shaft, and for the uncircumcised men the preputial cavity. The urethral meatus is not frequently involved, and if it is, the disease almost never extends beyond the fossa navicularis. Therefore, the eversion of the meatus or the use of a otoscope tip or pediatric nasal speculum is normally sufficient to appreciate the extent of the disease involvement. Perianal involvement in not common in heterosexual males, and usually reflects anal sexual play. Consequently, perianal warts are commonly encountered in homosexual males. Warts tend to be less common over the perineum, groin, pubic area, and scrotum. Given that the scrotum is frequently infected, it is clear that the development of a lesion is governed by local tissular factors yet to be identified.

In women, most warts are found over the posterior vestibule, including the fourchette, and the spread may extend toward the labia minora, the labia majora, and the clitoris. They can also be found on occasion over the perineum and the anus, but less often in the vagina, cervix, and urethra.

In a patient with genital warts, an anoscopic exam may be recommended if there are perianal warts, a history of anal receptive intercourse, or if the patient has anal symptoms. Intraanal warts typically do not extend beyond the pectinate line and a sigmoidoscopy is not necessary.

Immunosuppressed or immunodeficient (e.g., due to human immunodeficiency virus infection) patients tend to have more and larger lesions than an immunocompetent host. Because these patients are also prone to higher rates of anogenital cancers related to oncogenic HPV, it is important to look particularly for the presence of intraepithelial neoplasias and invasive cancers of the cervix and anus during the examination for genital warts. This includes, aside from the screening measures discussed elsewhere, a digital pelvic and anal examination, as well as the biopsy of any atypical or suspicious lesion.

Three quarters of patients with anogenital warts experience no symptoms other than noticing the presence of the lesions. Itching, burning, sometimes pain, tenderness or discomfort are the most common symptoms, which only rarely interfere with sexual intercourse. The psychological impact of the disease is responsible for the greatest burden in at least half of the patients. Patients express guilt, shame, anger, fear of transmission or infertility, concern for well-being, appearance, sexuality, and cure.

A recent large French study involving a representative sampling of 516 men and women with external genital warts demonstrated that at least 99% of genital warts are associated with an HPV infection. The decreasing order of prevalence was HPV type 6 (69%), 11 (16%), 16 (9%), 51 (8%), 52 (8%), 66 (6%), 53 (5%), 31 (3%), and 18 (3%). A third of the single lesions had multiple infections. The cumulative prevalence of HPV types 6 and 11 was 83%, and 88% for types 6, 11, 16, and 18.

3.1.2. Differential Diagnosis

Table 3.1 lists most conditions that might be confused with anogenital warts. Molluscum contagiosum (Fig. 3.5), another viral disease caused by a poxvirus, is frequently misidentified for warts. The lesions form sesssile, dome-shaped, round papules, with no pedunculation, and a color that is identical to the surrounding skin, but can be paler or redder due to inflammation. Their surface contour is smooth, with in most instances a telltale central dimple from which might be expressed a cheesy material containing viral particles. Molluscum contagiosum lesions tend to predominate over the pubis, extending over the lower abdomen, even over other parts of the body, rather than being present over the penis, scrotum, vulva, perinuem and anus. Acrochordons (skin tags) are benign, non-viral lesions that are also easy to confuse with warts, but they are soft, supple, non-keratinized, without disruption of the skin ridges. Moreover, they are typically less numerous than warts. Hirsutoid papillomatosis (see Table 3.1 for other synonyms) (Fig. 3.6) is a normal variant appearance of the base of the glans (corona glandis) characterized by the prominent development of

Table 3.1 *Differential Diagnosis of External Genital Warts*

External genital wart variant	Could be confused with
Papillomatous lesions	Molluscum contagiosum (C) Acrochordon (C) Condyloma latum (syphilis) (C, S) Hirsutoid papillomatosis/pearly coronal papules/ papillae corona glandis (C) Epidermoid cysts (C) Hidradenoma papilliferum (C, H) Pemphigus vegetans (C, H) Nodular scabies (C) Common warts (H) Intraepithelial neoplasia (H) Squamous cell carcinoma (H)
Giant lesions	Buschke-Löwenstein tumor (H) Squamous cell carcinoma (verrucous carcinoma) (H) Lymphogranuloma venereum (S)
Flat papules	Intraepithelial neoplasia (including Queyrat's erythroplasia) (H) Condyloma latum (S) Lichen planus (C, H) Lichen sclerosus et atrophicus (C, H) Lichen nitidus (C, H) Syringomas (C, H)
Pigmented lesions	Nevi (C, H) Seborrheic keratosis (C) Intraepithelial neoplasia (including bowenoid papulosis, Bowen's disease) (H)

Usual methods of diagnosis—C, clinical; H, histologic; S, serologic.

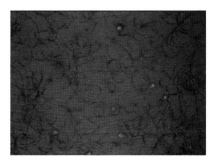

Figure 3.5 *Molluscum contagiosum on the pubis.*

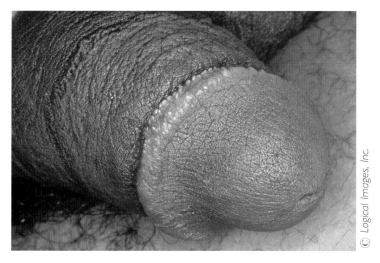

Figure 3.6 *Hirsutoid papillomatosis.*

papillae. It is recognized by the small size, pointed but smooth surface, and regular distribution of these papillae, which are also of a paler shade than the surrounding mucosa. In females, a similar variant of circumferential papillae may be encountered around the vaginal opening. A Buschke-Löwenstein tumor cannot be clinically differentiated from a giant condyloma. The histology shows features characteristic of condyloma acuminatum, but the exophytic and endophytic proliferation is prominent and this expansion may compromise the adjacent anatomic structures. Bowenoid papulosis, Bowen's disease, and erythroplasia of Queyrat are discussed in the next section.

3.2. Other Diseases of the Anogenital Tract

HPV can infect not only the penis, the vulva, and the perianal area, but also the anus, the vagina, and the cervix. This is one of the reasons why genital HPVs are also called mucosal HPVs. Exposure of these structures to HPV can lead to infection at many sites in the same patient, something referred as a "field effect". The resulting diseases range from condylomas (see the previous section for external genitalia condylomas) to carcinomas. Between these two opposite poles of severity are the precursor lesions to cancer that are called intraepithelial neoplasias. According to the site, one recognizes penile (PIN), vulvar (VIN), vaginal (VAIN), cervical (CIN), and anal (AIN) intraepithelial neoplasias. Another, older designation is *dysplasia*, even if unlike true dysplasia, these lesions are not the result of an abnormal embryologic development of the tissue. The definitive diagnosis is made by histology, and different grades of severity are recognized (see chap. 5). These lesions are squamous cell proliferations. In the case of the cervix, the HPV neoplastic process can affect either the squamous stratified epithelium and lead to squamous cell carcinoma, or less frequently the glandular epithelium, giving rise to adenocarcinoma and its precursor, adenocarcinoma in situ (AIS). In the cervix the diagnosis of these lesions can be established by both cytology and histology.

3.2.1. Condyloma

3.2.1.1. Cervical Condyloma (Flat Condyloma)

A cervical wart or condyloma results from the infection of the cervix with low-risk HPV types. It is diagnosed at the time of colposcopic evaluation for an abnormal Papanicolaou (Pap) smear (Fig. 3.7). A papillary-type cervical wart, which is rare and typically spares the transformation zone, is easy to see because exophytic. In contrast, a flat cervical condyloma may not be clinically evident on gross inspection of the cervix at the time of routine gynecologic examination. The subtle appearance of thickened, raised, and whitish epithelium can be easily concealed by cervical mucous. These warty lesions may present at multiple sites, affecting not only the

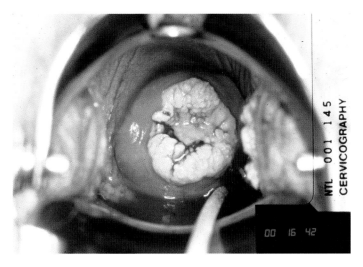

Figure 3.7 Cervical condyloma. Classic exophytic growth of cervical warts with the cervical os delineated by the presence of mucous (Courtesy of Richard Cherkis).

external cervix (exocervix), but potentially extending up into the cervical canal (endocervix) to the squamo-columnar junction.

3.2.1.2. Vaginal Condyloma

Vaginal warts may arise independently or in association with cervical and/or vulvar condyloma as an extension of disease. In immunocompromised individuals such as HIV-infected women, the extent of the vaginal condyloma can encompass the entire vaginal canal. Multifocal lesions are very common in these women and can make the diagnosis of more severe intraepithelial lesions difficult.

3.2.1.3. Anal Condyloma

Anal condyloma are usually recognized during the anoscopic examination as whitish papules that tend to be less exophytic than the perianal condylomas they are often accompanied by. Smaller lesions may require the application of 5% acetic acid for visualization and the use of a colposcope (so-called high-resolution anoscopy). Symptoms, if present, may include itching, discomfort, pain, and bleeding. A history of anal intercourse, use of anal insertive objects or fingers, and HIV infection should prompt an anoscopic examination combined with a digital rectal examination, especially if the patient has other anogenital HPV diseases.

3.2.2. Intraepithelial Neoplasia

3.2.2.1. Cervical Intraepithelial Neoplasia (CIN)

CIN is typically diagnosed during colposcopy (Fig. 3.8) (see chap. 5). This is a specialized technique. Because training and equipment are not readily available in the developing world, it is possible to use visual inspection aided by acetic acid (VIA) to detect CIN and effectively prevent cervical cancer, if not with the same accuracy that colposcopy allows. The incidence of CIN is increased in HIV-infected women, and the severity is correlated with the CD4+ T-cell count.

3.2.2.2. Vaginal Intraepithelial Neoplasia (VAIN)

VAIN like CIN is typically diagnosed during colposcopy. It tends to arise among patients in whom a previous or current diagnosis of cervical and/or vulvar dysplasia has been made. Occasionally, bleeding may be an early manifestation. Following hysterectomy, vaginal dysplasia can arise de novo and is associated with the same high-risk HPV types seen in cervical disease. Many of these women have disease detected from Pap smear surveillance following definitive treatment for their cervical dysplasia or cancer.

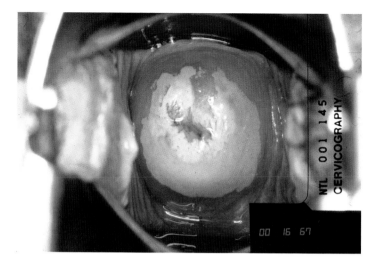

Figure 3.8 High grade cervical dysplasia within mild cervical change. Application of 3% acetic acid to the cervix reveals an internal border of acetowhite epithelium within the larger cervical lesion on colposcopic evaluation. This internal border delineates an area of higher grade dysplasia which is approaching the canal (Courtesy of Richard Cherkis).

3.2.2.3. Vulvar and Penile Intraepithelial Neoplasia (VIN and PIN)

Before VIN and PIN were recognized as such, two clinically characteristic variants had been identified, both predominantly associated with HPV-16 infection. One is bowenoid papulosis and the other is Bowen's disease. Bowenoid papulosis in its strictest definition is a clinical and histologic entity characterized by aggregated, multicentric papules, ranging in color from dark red to dark blue, while the cytoarchitecture is that of a condyloma with the histology of an intraepithelial neoplasia. It may transition to Bowen's disease, a carcinoma in situ that appears as a flat, scaly plaque, red to brown in color, an irregular surface contour, but with sharp borders. Erythroplasia of Queyrat is Bowen's disease confined to the glans penis. This nomenclature should be abandoned in favor of the broader VIN and PIN denomination (Fig. 3.9).

Nevertheless, due to the keratinized squamous epithelium of the vulva and penis, detection of premalignant changes can be difficult. Pruritus is the most classic symptom, but burning, bleeding, redness, swelling, and dyspareunia may also be present. Subtle asymmetric changes in pigmentation and texture of the vulvar skin should lead the clinician to perform a more in-depth inspection of the vulva and consider biopsy of affected tissue for pathologic diagnosis.

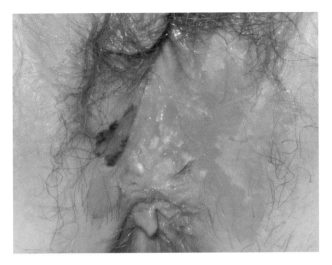

Figure 3.9 Vulvar intraepithelial neoplasia (VIN) with hyperhemic and hyperpigmented changes next to acetowhite epithelium (Courtesy of Brent DuBeshter).

3.2.2.3. Anal Intraepithelial Neoplasia (AIN)

The incidence of AIN, which is otherwise uncommon, is substantially raised by HIV infection and correlates with the level of immunosuppresion. The symptoms are similar to those of anal condylomas, and the evaluation of the patient is the same. As with the cervix, lesions can be detected by anal cytology, but it is high-resolution anoscopy (chaps. 5 and 6) combined with biopsy that permits the evaluation of lesions.

3.2.3. Invasive Carcinoma

Invasive carcinomas are the ultimate evolution of intraepithelial neoplasias, and except for when they are extensively invasive or metastatic, the clinical features are indistinguishable.

3.2.3.1. Cervical Carcinoma

Just as with CIN, the diagnosis of cervical cancer is usually made by cytology, colposcopy, and/or biopsy (Fig. 3.10). Most patients are asymptomatic. Those who have never been screened or deviate from recommended screening intervals are more likely to be symptomatic, most often with bleeding. These patients account for half the women who develop cervical cancer. Almost 90% of cervical cancers are squamous cell carcinomas, whereas 10% are adenocarcinomas, which are harder to detect early because

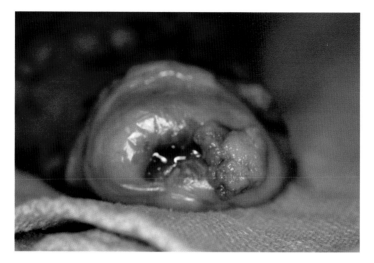

Figure 3.10 Squamous cell carcinoma of the cervix on hysterectomy specimen. Radical hysterectomy was performed for a Stage IB1 cervical carcinoma. The friable exophytic tumor mass on the cervix was first seen on work-up for post-coital bleeding.

they tend to arise from the endocervix. HPV-16 and HPV-18 account for about 70% of all cervical squamous cell carcinomas, while HPV-18 predominates over type 16 in the adenocarcinomas. In the HIV patient, cervical cancer is part of the case-definition for the acquired immunodeficiency syndrome (AIDS). This decision was made in anticipation because the severity of CIN seemed to correlate with the degree of immunosuppression, as measured by the CD4+ T-cell count. It is now clear that the incidence of cervical cancer is not affected by the degree of immunosuppression in HIV. Nevertheless, overall the incidence of cervical cancer is higher in the HIV population. Staging of cervical cancer follows the Fédération Internationale d'Obstétrique et Gynécologie (FIGO) nomenclature.

3.2.3.2. Vulvar Carcinoma

Vulvar cancer represents about 5% of all female malignancies, considerably less than cervical cancer. Squamous cell carcinoma of the vulva is also much less studied. Its clinical presentation, especially in the early stages, does not vary from that of VIN. Verrucous carcinoma is an exception because it is large and exophytic with a condylomatous appearance. There are different histologic variants (as with VIN), and these as well as age of the patients account for why HPV (mostly HPV-16) is associated with only 40% of vulvar cancers. HPV-associated cancers occur in younger patients and in lesions that have undifferentiated, warty or basaloid, features.

This remains one of the few reproductive tract cancers in which the TNM (tumor, nodal, metastasis) model is used. Microinvasion does not carry the same treatment implication as it does with cervical cancer, and therefore the determination of exact depth of invasion is inconsequential for anything greater than 1mm. If invasion is less than or equal to 1mm, the risk of lymph node metastasis is extremely low, and therefore the omission of a formal lymph node dissection is justified.

3.2.3.3. Vaginal Carcinoma

Similarly to preinvasive VAIN, the incidence of primary invasive vaginal carcinoma is extremely small, 1% to 2% of all lower genital tract cancers. Only 60% are associated with HPV infection by types 16 or 18. This subset of patients carry some of the same risk factors identified with cervical and vaginal cancer, namely number of sexual partners, early age of sexual debuts, smoking, and HPV seropositivity. Clinical staging is modeled after the paradigms already established for cervical and vulvar cancers, and follows the FIGO system.

3.2.3.4. Penile Carcinoma

Penile squamous carcinoma is a rare cancer, especially in the developed world. It arises from PIN, but the penile glans, the coronal sulcus, and the foreskin are areas of predilection. The lesions may be infiltrative, ulcerative, or proliferative; special examples of the latter are verrucous carcinomas and Buschke-Löwenstein tumors. The symptoms include itching, pain, bleeding, dyspareunia, foul odor, and discharge, which may be due to a fistulous tract. Like for the vulva, the undifferentiated histologic variants (warty, basaloid, and mixed) are the ones that have the highest association (70–100%) with high-risk HPV infection, with HPV-16 predominating. For the other types, the association is about 30%. Lack of neonatal circumcision has been identified as a strong risk factor, but other risk factors, such as hygiene, are probably involved since penile cancer is rare in the non-circumcised Nordic populations. Staging of this cancer is based on the TNM nomenclature.

3.2.3.5. Anal Carcinoma

Although anal cancer is a rare cancer in the general population, a history of anogenital warts, anal intercourse, and having sex with men are risk factors that are further magnified in the presence of an HIV infection, which increases the risk up to about 60-fold. Up to 90% of anal cancer are related to a high-risk HPV infection, with type 16 representing about 70% of all the types, and type 18 about 10%. In the early stages, the symptoms of anal cancer may be local and similar to those of AIN. Screening for anal cancer by cytology, digital rectal examination, anoscopic exam with or without the use of acetic acid or a colposcope will detect a large number of asymptomatic tumors that can be infiltrating, erosive, or fungating. Staging is done according to the TNM nomenclature.

3.3. Diseases of the Head and Neck Area and Other Sites

Warts can be present in any location of the mouth and oral cavity (Fig. 3.11). The clinical appearance is similar to that of genital warts, although on the mucous surfaces they may be flatter and hard to visualize in the absence of proper lighting. There are different histologic variants of oral warts, the most common is squamous cell papilloma (or squamous papilloma). The other variants are condyloma acuminatum, and verruca vulgaris. The first two are mostly associated with mucoso-genital HPV types 6, 11, and 16, whereas the last one is linked to cutaneous HPV types 2, 4, and 57. Focal epithelial hyperplasia (Heck's disease) is a benign condition of children and young adults, caused mostly by HPV types 13 and 32, which is found predominantly in Indian populations of the Americas. It presents as flesh-colored flat papules, sometimes confluent, that cover the mucosa of the oral cavity and buccal space. Although they may persist for several years, they eventually resolve spontaneously.

In recurrent respiratory papillomatosis, HPV-6 and -11, the main agents of genital warts, do cause laryngeal papillomas, a rare but serious and

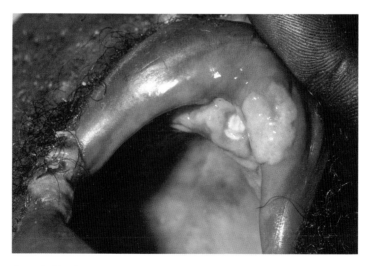

Figure 3.11 Oral warts on the lip and buccal mucosa.

potentially life-threatening disease due to the recurrent nature of the lesions and the risk of airway obstruction. Moreover, these otherwise benign papillomavirus types confer an oncogenic potential if these laryngeal papillomas extend to the lung or aerodigestive tract. Irradiation is strongly contra indicated as it promotes malignant transformation of the tumor. The disease has two forms of presentation, juvenile-onset, the more common, and adult-onset. An altered cry in the infant and voice hoarseness in the adult are the mode of presentation. The main risk factor for the juvenile form is exposure to an infected birth canal, whereas it is oral sex that is linked to the adult form of the disease.

Cancer of the oropharynx, which includes the lingual and palatine tonsils, is one of the most common forms of head and neck cancer. It is now well established that most of the cases are related to HPV-16 and -18 infections. Oral sex and marijuana uses are co-factors.

Nasal or sinonasal papillomatosis refers to a group of uncommon benign epithelial tumors of the sinonasal made of (a) exophytic papillomas, (b) inverted papillomas, and (c) columnar (oncocytic) cell papillomas. A majority of exophytic papillomas and a minority of inverted papillomas are associated with genital HPV types. HPV-16 has been identified in inverted papillomas that progressed to squamous cell carcinoma.

Although rare, HPV-16 has been associated with squamous cell carcinomas arising from the fingers periungueal area and from the conjunctive, especially in countries with high ultraviolet light.

Selected References
Web Sites

New York State Department of Health AIDS Institute. Available at: http://www.hivguidelines.org.
United States National Cancer Institute. Cancer treatment. Available at: http://www.cancer.gov.
World Health Organization. Available at: http://www.who.int/hpvcentre. Accessed September 2008.

Articles
External Genital Warts
Aubin F, Pretet JL, Jacquard AC, Saunier M, Carcopino X, Jaroud F, et al. Human papillomavirus genotype distribution in external acuminata condylomata: a Large French National Study (EDiTH IV). Clin Infect Dis 2008; 47:610–615.

Wiley DJ, Douglas J, Beutner K, Cox T, Fife K, Moscicki AB, et al. External genital warts: diagnosis, treatment, and prevention. Clin Infect Dis 2002; 35(suppl 2): S210–S224.

Cervix

Sellors JW, Sankaranarayanan R. Colposcopy and Treatment of Cervical Intraepithelial Neoplasia: A Beginners' Manual. Lyon: International Agency for Research on Cancer, 2003. Available at: http://screening.iarc.fr/doc/Colposcopymanual.pdf.

Long HJ 3rd, Laack NN, Gostout BS. Prevention, diagnosis, and treatment of cervical cancer. Mayo Clin Proc 1566; 82:1566–1574.

Moore DH. Cervical cancer. Obstet Gynecol 1152; 107:1152–1161.

Vulva and Vagina

Duong TH, Flowers LC. Vulvo-vaginal cancers: risks, evaluation, prevention and early detection. Obstet Gynecol Clin North Am 2007; 34:783–802.

Penis

Bleeker MC, Heideman DA, Snijders PJ, Horenblas S, Dillner J, Meijer CJ. Penile cancer: epidemiology, pathogenesis and prevention. World J Urol 2008. Accessed November 18, 2008.

Anus

Eng C. Anal cancer: current and future methodology. Cancer Invest 2006; 24: 535–544.

Oral Cavity and Head and Neck

Bonnez W. Editorial comment: issues with HIV and oral human papillomavirus infections.[comment]. AIDS Reader 2002; 12(4):174–176.

Gillison ML. Current topics in the epidemiology of oral cavity and oropharyngeal cancers. Head Neck 2007; 29:779–792.

D'Souza G, Kreimer AR, Viscidi R, Pawlita M, Fakhry C, Koch WM, et al. Case-control study of human papillomavirus and oropharyngeal cancer. N Engl J Med 2007; 356:1944–1956.

HIV

Bratcher J, Palefsky J. Anogenital human papillomavirus coinfection and associated neoplasia in HIV-positive men and women. The PRN Notebook 2008; 12(9). Available at: www.prn.org. Accessed November 2008.

Patel P, Hanson DL, Sullivan PS, Novak RM, Moorman AC, Tong TC, et al. Incidence of types of cancer among HIV-infected persons compared with the general population in the United States, 1992–2003. Ann Intern Med 2008; 148:728–736.

Treatment

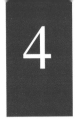

William Bonnez

Infectious Diseases Division, Department of
Medicine, University of Rochester School of
Medicine and Dentistry, Rochester, New York,
U.S.A.

Eugene P. Toy

Gynecologic Oncology, Department of Obstetrics
and Gynecology, University of Rochester School
of Medicine and Dentistry, Rochester, New York,
U.S.A.

There is no treatment to eradicate HPV infections at the moment. Therefore, the goal of treatment is to eliminate or control the diseases that results from the HPV infection by destruction of the lesions by physico-chemical means, or by induction of an inflammatory or immune response. The great variety of approaches that exist reflects the fact that there is still no uniformly safe and consistently effective treatment for these lesions. Many of these therapies have been developed empirically (Table 4.1).

4.1. The Treatment Modalities

4.1.1. Chemical Methods

4.1.1.1. Acids

Trichloroacetic acid (TCA) and to a lesser extent bichloroacetic acid as a 50% to 90% solution are particularly favored by gynecologists. These cauterizing and keratolytic agents are predominantly used for the treatment of warts on mucosal surfaces such as the non-hairy vulva and the anal canal. The application with a cotton swab is painful. Ulceration and scabbing are not uncommon. For this reason great care should be exercised so that the acid does not run over the surrounding healthy skin. If it does, it can be neutralized with sodium bicarbonate or talcum powder. Comparative trials of these treatment modalities are lacking.

> *- TCA (e.g., Tri-Chlor; 15-mL bottle): 50% to 90% solution applied to the lesion weekly, up to six times.*

Table 4.1 Anogenital Warts Treatment Responses

Treatment modality	Complete response rate (%)	Relapse rates (%)
TCA	64–83	55
Podophyllin	35–51	60–85
Podofilox	57–72	32–50
Interferon (intralesional)	40–52	18–37
Imiquimod	35–61	13
Kunecatechins	57	
Cold-blade surgery	87–94	20–31
Electrosurgery	58–94	22
Cryosurgery	64–76	19–40
Laser surgery	93–99	49–65

These rates are derived from various studies, not all comparative, controlled, or randomized. Furthermore, variations in study design, length and method of follow-up, and sex of the subjects are additional limitations to making any comparisons.

4.1.1.2. Antimitotics and Antimetabolites

4.1.1.2.1. Podophyllin and podofilox   For the last 50 years of the past century, podophyllin was probably the most common treatment of genital warts. It is made from the rhizome of *Podophyllum peltatum*, or also, outside North America, the more potent *Podophyllum emodi*, and usually prepared in a benzoin tincture as 25% podophyllum (USP). Lignans in the compound are responsible for the anti-wart activity as well as the toxicity. The most active of these lignans is podophyllotoxin, which in its purified form is now known as podofilox, a compound available as a 0.5% solution or gel. The main mode of action results from the binding to tubulin and the disruption of the mitotic spindle polymerization, thus causing the arrest of cell division.

Podophyllotoxin and podofilox are toxic. Among the local adverse reactions itching, pain, inflammation, erosions or ulcerations, bleeding, and burns are noted in decreasing frequency from 17% to 1% of patients. Severe reactions may lead to scarring. A contact dermatitis to benzoin or guaiacumwood may occur with podophyllum. Application of these preparations for more than 24 hours or on the healthy skin should be strictly avoided, because systemic absorption through the tegument, especially with podophyllin, may cause nausea and vomiting, and less frequently neuropathy, coma, even death. Bone marrow and renal toxicities are also possible.

The treatment also temporarily disturbs lesion histology. In particular the abnormal mitotic figures may lead to the erroneous diagnosis of intra-epithelial neoplasia. Podofilox offers a better toxicity and potency stability profile than podophyllin, and is strongly preferred for the treatment of genital warts. The ability to be administered by the patient is another substantial advantage of podofilox over podophyllin.

When compared to each other for efficacy, podofilox has been at least equivalent to podophyllin, which itself has been inferior to cryotherapy, electrosurgery, or excisional surgery. There does not appear to be any difference in efficacy between the solution or gel formulation of podofilox; however, the gel has the advantage of not running off as easily as the solution on the healthy skin. Podofilox is superior to placebo for the treatment of genital warts, and is effective at preventing recurrence as long as it is applied, at least for 8 weeks. Both podophyllin and podofilox are contraindicated during pregnancy and not more than a 10 cm^2 area should be treated at one time.

- ***Podophyllin*** *(e.g., Podocon-25, Podofin; 15-mL bottle): 25% in benzoin solution applied weekly to the lesion, up to six times.*
- ***Podofilox*** *(Condylox; 3.5-mL bottle or 3.5-g tube): 0.5% solution or gel self applied twice a day for three days per week, for up to four weeks.*

4.1.1.2.2. 5-Fluorouracil (5-FU)

5-FU is a pyrimidine analog that blocks the synthesis of DNA and to a lesser extent RNA. It is available as a 1% (Fluoroplex) and 5% (Efudex) cream. It has many empiric indications in dermatology, including for the treatment of genital warts. Its efficacy is difficult to establish, but appears to be similar to that of podophyllin. It is reportedly quite effective for intra-meatal warts. Its application is associated with pain, itching, burning, erosions, hyperpigmentation, and when applied in the vagina it may cause adenosis, or possibly vaginal clear cell carcinoma. 5-FU has bone marrow toxicity and cannot be considered safe during pregnancy.

4.1.1.2.3. Indole-3-carbinole (I3C) and diindolyl methane (DIM)

I3C and its main active metabolite, DIM, are two compounds found in cruciferous vegetables (broccoli, cabbage, cauliflower, …) that activate the 2-hydroxylation of estradiol leading to the formation of 2-hydroxyestrone instead of 16-α-hydroxyestrone, a derivative that stimulates HPV-induced proliferation. I3C (Indoplex) is used as food supplement in the management of respiratory papillomas, and was shown to be superior to placebo for the treatment of CIN 2 or 3.

> **- DIM** *(Phytosorb-DIM Capsules; 150-mg capsule, 60 capsules per bottle, or 75-mg capsule, 90 capsules per bottle): one oral daily dose of 5 to 8 mg/kg/day.*

4.1.1.3. Interferon, Immunomodulators, Antivirals, and Others

Interferons (α, β, and γ), with the exception of the new pegylated formulations, have been extensively and rigorously evaluated for the treatment of genital warts. Only when used intralesionally have they been consistently active. However, their modest activity when compared to placebo, their cost, and the limited number of lesions that can be treated by the intralesional route have been significant limitations to their broad use. Furthermore, systemic side-effects, which are typically limited to fever, chills, malaise, myalgias and, headaches can be troublesome. Even if they tend to abate significantly and rapidly with time, they can be troublesome. Interferons are contra-indicated during pregnancy.

> **- Interferon** *(e.g., Intron A, Alferon N): 1 million units injected three times weekly directly into one to all lesions for three to eight weeks.*

4.1.1.3.1. Imiquimod
Imiquimod is an imidazoquinoline that induces the local production of interferon α and other cytokines. Available as a 5% cream (Aldara) it is approved for the self-treatment of external genital warts, but it also has been used with success for the treatment of internal anogenital warts and of intraepithelial neoplasias of the anus, vulva, and vagina. Warts located in moist areas tend to respond better that those located on dry skin, and this explains the approximately two-fold greater efficacy in women than men. Local side-effects are common, but usually well-tolerated. They include itching, burning sensation, redness, erosion, and edema. Length of treatment, up to 16 weeks, and its related cost are two disadvantages of Aldara. It should not be used during pregnancy.

> **- Imiquimod** *(Aldara box of 12 single use 250-mg packets): 5% cream applied at bedtime, three times a week, every other day, for at least 8 weeks and up to 16 weeks.*

4.1.1.3.2. Cimetidine
Cimetidine an H_2-blocker has immunomodulatory effects in vitro that have led to its use for the treatment of genital warts. However, randomized controlled trials have failed to demonstrate efficacy.

4.1.1.3.3. Cidofovir Cidofovir is acyclic nucleotide notable for its inhibition of the DNA polymerase of herpesviruses. A 1% gel (not commercially available) has shown superiority to placebo for genital warts treatment. The mechanism of action does not involve the blockade of a DNA polymerase that HPV does not have; instead, cidofovir appears to enhance the death of HPV-infected keratinocytes by apoptosis. Side-effects include pain, erosions and ulcerations. Cidofovir has also been used topically or intralesionally for the treatment of recurrent respiratory papillomatosis, aerodigestive tumors, VIN, and CIN.

4.1.1.3.4. Veregen Veregen is the latest addition to the therapeutic armamentarium. This is a 15% ointment of kunecatechins, compounds that are obtained by partial purification of a water extract of green tea (*Camellia sinensis*). Epigallocatechin gallate is the most abundant compound. The mode of action is not clearly established. When compared to placebo, Veregen has shown superior efficacy for the self-treatment of external genital warts. The recommended duration of treatment and the side-effects are similar to those of imiquimod, but the need for thrice daily application and a red color that may stain underwear are substantial inconveniences. It should not be used during pregnancy.

> *- **Kunecatechins** (Veregen; 15-g tube): 15% ointment applied three times a day for up to 16 weeks.*

4.1.2. Physical Methods

All the physical methods require an operator.

4.1.2.1. Cold-Blade Excision

The removal of genital warts with scissors or a scalpel, under local anesthesia, is a very effective therapeutic approach, especially when the lesions are easily accessible and their number limited. Scarring is usually not a problem. The development of microresectors has facilitated the excision of laryngeal papillomas. Scalpel conization of the cervix, progressively replaced since the 1980's by electrosurgical techniques, has been for a long-time the main approach for the treatment of CIN. Cold-blade excision is ideal if the margin status of frankly invasive cancerous tissue is important for review.

4.1.2.2. Electrosurgery

Different techniques based on the use of electricity to cut, burn, or vaporize tissue make up electrosurgery. They are called electrosection, electrocautery, electrocoagulation, electrofulguration, and electrodesiccation. Their nomenclature is not firmly established, but varies according to the number of electrodes used, contact with the tissue, shape of the current wave form, amperage and voltage. Electrocoagulation and electro-dessication have been mostly used for genital warts. Application before the procedure of EMLA cream, a topical anesthetic containing prilocaine and lidocaine, provides good pain control. Scarring may occur. Large loop excision of the transformation zone (LLETZ), also called loop electro-surgical excision procedure (LEEP), is the procedure of choice for the treatment of CIN. This can be done under local anesthesia. These proce-dures increase the risk of preterm delivery. Some of the electrosurgery techniques do not destroy the tissue sample and histology can be reviewed. However, the margins may not interpretable due to cautery artifact.

4.1.2.3. Cryotherapy, Heat Therapy, and Ultrasound

The spraying of liquid nitrogen (boiling temperature $-196°C$) is a popular treatment method for anogenital warts. The spray nozzle is directed to the lesion and the cryogenic released for about 20 seconds to generate in the tissue an ice ball that extends slightly, about 1 mm, beyond the lesion. A second freezing may be applied immediately after thawing. Treatment is typically applied weekly up to six times. Pain is initially stinging in nature, but brief in duration, the time for the nerve endings to freeze. It is replaced by a discomfort upon thawing of the tissues. Once the procedure is over, the discomfort is usually minimal and not incapacitating. Local anesthesia is rarely needed, but can be achieved with the application of the EMLA cream. Scarring is unusual. The same technique can be used for intra-epithelial neoplasias of the external anogenital tract or for vaginal warts and intraepithelial neoplasias.

Cryotherapy is also used for the treatment of cervical condylomas and CIN. It is typically delivered by direct contact with a cryoprobe through which circulates carbon dioxide (boiling temperature, $-78.5°C$) or nitrous oxide (boiling temperature, $-89.5°C$). It is a procedure of choice for pregnant patients.

Heat has been used, if less frequently than cold, to treat HPV diseases. An infrared coagulator has been effective destroying external genital warts (about 80% complete response). This instrument also has become a tool of choice for the treatment of anal HPV diseases, from benign to high-grade intraepithelial neoplasia, especially in the HIV seropositive population. Another instrument, the cold coagulator, which is a teflon-coated probe that can be heated from $60°C$ to $100°C$ while applied to the tissue has been effective for the eradication of CIN.

Ultrasound can produce a phenomenon called acoustic cavitation, which is the rapid, oscillatory formation and collapse of microbubbles in tissue resulting in intense thermal variation and chemical reactions. This can be used to destroy lesions. This approach, called cavitronic ultrasonographic aspiration (CUSA) has been used for HPV-associated vulvar and vaginal diseases.

4.1.2.4. Laser Therapy

Lasers produce a high-energy, collimated light beam. This light is monochromatic and the wavelength determines the specific medical application. The CO_2 laser is the instrument of choice for the treatment of mucosogenital lesion because its infrared light ($\lambda = 10,600$ nm) vaporizes the intratissular water. By varying the focus of the beam the operator can either cut or vaporize the lesions. Further control is applied on how the light is emitted, either continuously or intermittently. Operator skill is important and undoubtedly contributes to the varying outcomes that have been reported in uncontrolled studies. Laser surgery is applicable to the treatment of external and internal anogenital warts—including during pregnancy—intraepithelial neoplasias, especially of the cervix, and recurrent respiratory papillomatosis. Pain is significant and local, sometimes general, anesthesia is necessary. The EMLA cream is an effective topical anesthetic for laser surgery. Up to a quarter of patients experience pain, bleeding, swelling, and scarring after the procedure.

Photodynamic laser therapy is a specialized technique whereby a photosensitizing compound is preferentially delivered either topically or systemically to the HPV lesions, which are then irradiated with a laser of the proper wavelength to activate the compound, and achieve lesion destruction. It has been used for genital warts, but more so for the management of recurrent respiratory papillomatosis.

4.1.3. Therapeutic Vaccines

Although efforts are already devoted to the development of therapeutic vaccines, none are currently on the market. Among the various approaches in different stages of clinical development two ought to be mentioned. The first is the ZYC101a vaccine that is delivered intramuscularly in biodegradable microparticles that contain a DNA plasmid encoding HLA-A2-restricted sequences of HPV-16 E7 as well as HPV-18 E6 and E7 sequences. In a phase II study it led to the regression of CIN2 or three lesions, but only in women younger than 25 years. The second vaccine is HspE7, a fusion protein made of bacillus Calmette-Guérin heat shock protein 65 as adjuvant and an HPV-16 polypeptide. In preliminary, uncontrolled studies this vaccine, which is administered subcutaneously, has shown some efficacy for the treatment of genital warts and AIN in HIV seropositive patients, and recurrent respiratory papillomatosis.

4.1.4. Suggestion, Hypnosis, and Homeopathy

There is no solid evidence that suggestion, hypnosis, or homeopathy are effective for the treatment of HPV diseases.

4.2. Approach to Treatment

Therapy is directed at HPV-associated diseases not infections, for which no reliable therapeutic solutions exist. The treatment of most HPV diseases is not rigorously codified, and no one modality is optimal. This is the consequence of the limited availability of appropriate comparative therapeutic trials. Therefore, in spite of the existence of guidelines for the approach of some HPV diseases, personal experience and instrument availability play an important role in the selection a particular treatment modality. Unfortunately for the patient, treatment costs can vary greatly.

4.2.1. External Anogenital Warts

The reasons to treat genital warts include the restoration of normal physical appearance and psychological well-being, the relief of the symptoms, and the opening an obstructed birth canal. Whether this impacts on HPV transmission, which is likely, or on the rare progression to malignancy is unknown. The decision to treat should be balanced with the knowledge that up to 20% of patients with genital warts will have a spontaneous resolution within three to four months, and that treatments are costly, and have potential complications.

No treatment offers the assurance of a complete and durable response, but with the possible exception of a long disease duration, the predictors of a poor response are not well-known. It is usually not advocated to evaluate the partner, but this may be important for reassurance, risk education, and the prevention of other sexually transmitted diseases. There is evidence that condom use should be encouraged during the treatment period and afterwards to improve treatment response and prevent re-infection (see chap. 7).

Table 4.1 provides estimates of the efficacy of the main treatment modalities of genital warts. The following is a general summary of the clinical evidence that may direct the selection of a particular treatment modality. Cryotherapy, electrosurgery, cold-blade excision, and podofilox are superior to podophyllin. Podophyllin is more likely to cause adverse reactions than podofilox. Cryotherapy, electrosurgery, and TCA have probably equivalent efficacy. Intralesional interferon, but probably not systemic interferon is superior to placebo, but only a limited number of lesions can be treated. Cost and tolerability limit this treatment to few, large, recalcitrant, life-threatening lesions. Cost may limit laser surgery to second line therapy, but it may be useful when lesions are numerous and recalcitrant.

Self-administration makes podofilox and imiquimod, which is likely more effective, desirable treatment options. Veregen (kunecatechins ointment) is approved, but not yet distributed in the United States. It is likely to become a third option for self-treatment. Self-treatment has the drawback of frequent applications for many weeks. Some patients desire a more expeditive approach, in which case TCA and cryotherapy are two simple and effective options. If the number of warts is limited, one should consider scissor excision, which give excellent results. Urethral warts may be treated with podofilox, cryotherapy, or less likely with podophyllin or 5-FU.

Other types of treatment such as cidofovir, which is very expensive, should be reserved for recalcitrant cases. Although there might be valid reasons why a different treatment modality should be used in case of failure, there is no evidence that change is necessary given that complete response may still occur after a treatment repeat.

TCA, cryotherapy, cold-blade surgery, electrosurgery, and laser surgery can be used in the pregnant patient. In the immunocompromised host, including HIV patients, treatments are generally about half as effective. Therefore, disease control rather than eradication may be at time the only attainable objective. Minimizing the side-effects of cumulative treatments becomes very important.

4.2.2. Other Diseases of the Genital Tract

Treatment of related sequelae from HPV infection is reserved for disease states in which there is a significant risk of malignant transformation or when quality of life is significantly impaired. The large majority of lesions related to HPV infection will resolve over time or remain stable. The ability for these disease states to revert to normal relies largely on an intact immune system. While ablative therapies can halt the progression of current disease, definitive treatment may be necessary in individuals at high risk of malignant progression.

4.2.2.1. Condylomas

4.2.2.1.1. Cervical condyloma (flat condyloma) Cervical warts or flat condyloma generally behave indolently in spite of the potential for multifocality. The most common course of treatment is expectant management unless there is concomitant intraepithelial neoplasia. Given that women most commonly affected with cervical warts are in their 20s, the majority will be subsequently clear the lesions spontaneously and have no future sequelae from their warts. If necessary, ablative therapies with cryotherapy (freezing) of the cervix and laser ablation can be performed in cases of persistent, symptomatic disease.

4.2.2.1.2. Vaginal condyloma The elimination of vaginal warts can be challenging due to the potential for multifocality with limited access to redundant portions of the vaginal mucosa. TCA and many of the surgical methods used for the treatment of vulvar condyloma such as laser ablation and CUSA and are also employed. The difficulty lies in the degree of exposure to the many folds of the vaginal wall which can leave portions of the condyloma inaccessible and undertreated. This limited access combined with the propensity for these lesions to recur in immunocompromised individuals requires more of a maintenance therapy rather than definitive removal.

4.2.2.2. Intraepithelial Neoplasias

4.2.2.2.1. Cervical intraepithelial neoplasia (CIN) The natural course of CIN is over the span of several years with spontaneous regression of the majority of incident cases. The risk of progression of the most severe of cervical dysplasias, squamous cell carcinoma in situ, to invasive carcinoma is only about 30% when left untreated. Regression rates of less severe disease such as CIN1 and CIN2 are as high as 65% and 50%, respectively. When the diagnosis of severe dysplasia of the cervix is being evaluated, removal of the affected tissue is necessary to rule out carcinoma as well as treat the affected area. This too can be achieved with surgical techniques that provide a pathologic specimen as well as those that serve solely to ablate the tissue involved. Although margin status is not useful in predicting the risk of recurrence for preinvasive disease or progression to carcinoma, it can guide the clinician in recommendations for definitive treatment of microinvasive carcinoma (see below).

Of the ablative techniques that provide tissue by which the pathologist can analyze the severity of disease, the LEEP conization of the cervix is the most commonly used technique by which the affected portion of the cervix is removed (Table 4.2). Cold knife conization is preferred for certain lesions that are not amenable to the curvature or size of the wire loop used for the LEEP procedure. The other advantage to using the scalpel or knife for excision is the avoidance of thermal artifact at the margin of excision, which can be important in the interpretation of adequacy of treatment for microinvasive disease.

Table 4.2 *Management of Genital Intraepithelial Neoplasias*

Primary Site	Grade[a]	Surgical	Medical
Cervix	1	Cryotherapy	Observe with serial Pap smears
	2 & 3	LEEP Cold-knife conization	Non-applicable
Vulva	1	Cold-knife	Observe with serial colposcopy 1% 5-FU[b] cream
	2 & 3	Cold-knife Laser CUSA[c]	1% 5-FU cream
Vagina	1	Laser	Observe with serial Pap smears 5% 5-FU cream
	2 & 3	Cold-knife Laser CUSA	5% 5-FU cream

[a]These recommendations may no necessarily apply to carcinomas in situ.
[b]5-FU, 5-fluorouracil.
[c]CUSA, cavitronic ultrasonographic cavitation.

4.2.2.2.2. Vulvar intraepithelial neoplasia (VIN) Treatment of VIN3 is paramount because this lesion has a higher rate of progression to invasive cancer than CIN3 (Table 4.2). Lesions that progress quickly and have characteristics of invasive growth should be excised to rule out carcinoma. CUSA can also provide tissue for pathologic submission. To maximize the chance of cure, laser ablation in non-hair bearing regions should be performed to a depth of 1 to 2 mm while hair-bearing regions with follicles present require a greater depth of treatment to 2 to 3 mm. Topical agents such as 5-FU cream have been used but can cause skin reactions in those with hypersensitivity. A concentration of 1% 5-FU cream (Fluoroplex) is used sparingly to affected areas either on consecutive weekdays for 2 weeks or once a week for up to 12 weeks at a time.

4.2.2.2.3. Vaginal intraepithelial neoplasia (VAIN) The most common area affected by VAIN is the vaginal apex. Access to the vaginal canal and all of its rugations contained within can be difficult. When surgical options are exhausted, topical treatment with 5-FU has been utilized to treat the canal in its entirety (Table 4.2). A concentration of 5% 5-FU (Efudex) cream is self-administered intravaginally via an applicator once a week at bedtime for up to 12 weeks at a time.

4.2.2.3. Invasive Carcinoma

Treatment of invasive carcinoma of the lower genital tract is dependent upon stage and the extent of surgical resectability (see the National Cancer Institute Web site). Early microinvasion of the cervix can be managed with more conservative surgical treatment.

4.2.3. Diseases of the Anal Canal

Anecdotes and short series strengthened by opinion are for the most part the basis for most therapeutic approaches for anal HPV benign and premalignant lesions. They include the use of TCA or imiquimod, but also 5-FU cream and retinoids. However, physical methods are often used, including cold blade surgery, cryotherapy, electrosurgery, and laser surgery. The significant rise in anal HPV-associated lesions and cancer in the HIV population has stimulated the development of a more rigorous approach. The infrared coagulator has received particular attention, and seems to be versatile and effective. In the HIV population, biopsies of lesions are recommended, and treatment is primarily directed to AIN2 and 3, which offer the greatest risk of evolution to invasive cancer. The complete response rate is about half for most lesions. AIN1 and benign lesions are usually observed carefully because treatment yields only modest complete response rates, and treatment has costs in side-effects and money that are better reserved for more severe conditions. Anal cancer is treated according to stage with radiation or radiation plus chemotherapy (5-FU, mitomycin, cis-platinum, …). Surgery is no longer the first line treatment except when small lesions are present (see National Cancer Institute Web site).

4.2.4. Diseases of the Head and Neck Area

Oral warts are usually treated with any of the physical ablation methods (laser, cold-blade, cryotherapy, electrosurgery). Podophyllin has also been used.

The management goal of recurrent respiratory papillomatosis is maintaining a free airway. This is achieved using laser surgery, which is delicate because of the risk of scarring. Cold blade surgery is also used, in particular using a microdebrider. An early disease onset is associated with a higher number of surgical interventions. Adjuvant therapies are commonly used, most commonly with I3C or DIM, interferon, photodynamic therapy, and cidofovir. Other adjuvant modalities with no more than anecdotal evidence of efficacy are also employed such as acyclovir, retinoids, and mumps vaccine injection.

The management of cancers of the oral cavity, oropharynx, and nasopharynx is too complex to be summarized here, but it relies of the three main oncologic treatment modalities: surgery, radiation, and chemotherapy.

Selected References

Web Sites

New York State Department of Health AIDS Institute. Available at: http://www. hivguidelines.org.

United States National Cancer Institute. Cancer treatment. Available at: http://www. cancer.gov.

Articles and Books

Buck HW Jr. Warts (genital). BMJ Clin Evid 2007; 12(1602):1–20.

Derkay CS, Darrow DH. Recurrent respiratory papillomatosis. Ann Otol Rhinol Laryngol 2006; 115:1–11.

Lacey CJ. Therapy for genital human papillomavirus-related disease. J Clin Virol 2005; 32(suppl 1):S82–S90.

Melnikow J, Nuovo J, Willan AR, Chan BK, Howell LP. Natural history of cervical squamous intraepithelial lesions: a meta-analysis. Obstet Gynecol 1998; 92:727–735.

Sellors JW, Sankaranarayanan R. Colposcopy and Treatment of Cervical Intraepithelial Neoplasia: A Beginners' Manual. Lyon: International Agency for Research on Cancer, 2003. Available at: http://screening.iarc.fr/doc/Colposcopymanual.pdf.

Snoeck R. Papillomavirus and treatment. Antivir Res 2006; 71(2–3):181–191.

Workowski KA, Berman SM. Sexually transmitted diseases treatment guidelines, 2006. MMWR Recomm Rep 2006; 55(RR-11):1–94. Available at: http://www. cdc.gov/std/treatment/2006/rr5511.pdf.

Wright TC Jr., Massad LS, Dunton CJ, Spitzer M, Wilkinson EJ, Solomon D. 2006 consensus guidelines for the management of women with cervical intraepithelial neoplasia or adenocarcinoma in situ. Am J Obstet Gynecol 2007; 197:340–345. Available at: http://www.asccp.org/pdfs/consensus/algorithms_hist_07.pdf.

Wright TC Jr., Massad LS, Dunton CJ, Spitzer M, Wilkinson EJ, Solomon D. 2006 consensus guidelines for the management of women with abnormal cervical cancer screening tests. Am J Obstet Gynecol 2007; 197:346–355. Available at: http://www.asccp.org/pdfs/consensus/algorithms_hist_07.pdf.

Diagnosis

Eugene P. Toy
Gynecologic Oncology, Department of Obstetrics
and Gynecology, University of Rochester School
of Medicine and Dentistry, Rochester, New York,
U.S.A.

Mark H. Stoler
Division of Surgical Pathology, Department of
Pathology, University of Virginia Health System,
Charlottesville, Virginia, U.S.A.

Patti E. Gravitt
Departments of Epidemiology and Molecular
Microbiology and Immunology, Johns Hopkins
Bloomberg School of Public Health, Baltimore,
Maryland, U.S.A.

Robert C. Rose
Infectious Diseases Division, Departments of
Medicine, and Microbiology and Immunology,
University of Rochester School of Medicine and
Dentistry, Rochester, New York, U.S.A.

The majority of external anogenital lesions caused by HPV are warts for which the diagnosis is clinical, and typically warts do not require ancillary diagnosis methods. However, for many of the internal HPV-associated lesions, especially if they carry a risk of neoplasia, the naked eye is not sufficient to establish a diagnosis for proper management. In this chapter, the techniques that aid to the diagnosis at the organ, tissue, cellular, and molecular levels are reviewed.

5.1. Colposcopy

Cervical adenocarcinoma and squamous cell carcinoma are preceded by the abolition of normal maturation and differentiation patterns. Colposcopy is the examination using magnifying optics (the colposcope) of the cervix, and by extension of lower genital tract tissues to identify these areas of aberrant differentiation. Enhancing the visualization, the application of 3–5% acetic acid or white vinegar acts as a mucolytic and causes, by a mechanism that is not well-understood, the whitening of the tissues that have abnormal

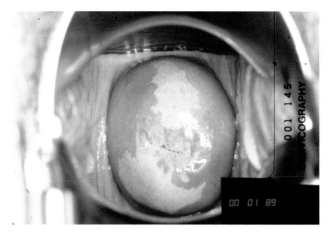

Figure 5.1 Acetowhite change of the cervical epithelium. A "geographic" distribution of acetowhite epithelial change after application of 3% acetic acid to the cervix is shown indicating low-grade cervical dysplasia.

nuclear to cytoplasmic ratio. The more severely abnormal lesions will require more time to produce acetowhitening, but ultimately the changes will be more pronounced (Fig. 5.1). These color changes guide the clinician to obtain biopsies from the most suspicious areas. Table 5.1 details the colposcopic nomenclature and a lesion classification scheme.

Colposcopy and inspection of other sites with the use of a colposcope suffer from limited accuracy, as well as limited inter- and intra-observer agreement. This is why the biopsy of abnormal appearing tissue is a complement to these techniques.

5.1.1. Cervical Intraepithelial Neoplasia (CIN)

With cell changes that occur by the process of *metaplasia*, the normal gross appearance of the cervix can be mistaken for a neoplastic process. Application of 3% acetic acid allows for the identification of abnormal maturation indicative of dysplasia distinguishing it from areas of metaplasia (see chap. 6). In addition to acetic acid, some colposcopists will perform a complementary test called Schiller's test with the application of an iodine-based solution called Lugol's solution. The normal areas of glycogen-containing cells will stain a mahogany brown while dysplastic or carcinomatous tissue will be "Schiller-negative" (Fig. 5.2A, B). This test is non-specific and metaplastic tissue can also be negative. Therefore, this test cannot be used alone.

Table 5.1 Colposcopic Scoring System

	Score			
	0	**1**	**2**	**3**
Color	Low intensity, semitransparent, insdistinct	Shiny, gray-white, intermediate	Dull, oyster-white, gray	Yellow, necrotic, friable
Margins	Microcondylomatous, micropapillary, indistinct, feathered, flocculated, angular, jagged	Regular, symmetrical, smooth	Rolled, peeling edges, internal borders	Exophytic, nodular, ulcerated
Mosaicism, punctation	Fine	None	Coarse	

The higher the score the highest is the likelihood of neoplasia. This scoring system is derived for the Reid and Scalzi scheme. *Source:* Massad LS, Jeronimo J, Schiffman M. Interobserver agreement in the assessment of components of colposcopic grading. Obstet Gynecol 2008; 111:1279–1284.

TERMINOLOGY

Acetowhite epithelium (AWE): With the application of acetic acid, the characteristic whitish appearance of the epithelial surface which can indicate dysplastic change.

Borders: A geographic delineation of dysplastic epithelium reflecting an atypical growth process.

Punctation: The protrusion of capillaries at the surface of the epithelium.

Mosaicism: A system of capillaries that form septations giving a "honeycomb" appearance to the surface of the epithelium.

Atypical vessels: Bizarre branching of vessels which may also be of larger caliber than usually seen at the surface of the tissue.

Satisfactory colposcopy: When the entire squamo-columnar junction is visible (see screening) and the extent of dysplastic lesions are seen in full.

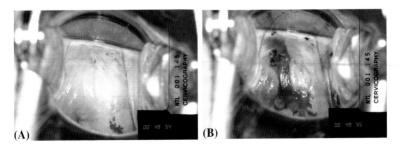

(A) (B)

Figure 5.2 (**A**) *Acetowhite change of the vaginal epithelium. A localized lesion in the left fornix of the vagina is seen after application of 3% acetic acid. Mild punctuation indicative of dysplasia can also be appreciated. (**B**) Schiller's negative test. The same vaginal lesion after application of Lugol's iodine solution showing lack of uptake consistent with the diagnosis of vaginal dysplasia.*

5.1.2. Vaginal Intraepithelial Neoplasia (VAIN)

Acetowhite change from VAIN is difficult to see when the folds of the vagina are redundant. Careful inspection of *all* the vaginal walls is necessary to assess disease. One uses a wide-billed (e.g., Graves) speculum, and inserts the blades to the full extent of the vagina. The inspection is conducted while slowly pulling out the speculum. When this type of speculum is used in younger, parous women with a more distensible vagina, it may fail to give adequate exposure. It may be then necessary to use a sidewall speculum or tongue depressor in addition to the anterior/posterior blades of the Graves' speculum in order to view subtle sidewall lesions.

5.1.3. Vulvar Intraepithelial Neoplasia (VIN)

The normal pigmentation changes that occur with aging and loss of estrogen production can be mistaken for dysplasia. Hypopigmentation seen grossly can be indicative of evolving dysplasia especially if isolated assymetrically distributed. Application of 5% acetic acid for a full two to three minutes is required due to the keratinization of the vulvar skin. Acetowhite lesions can then be examined under the colposcope, and areas that would otherwise display a normal physiologic loss of skin elasticity can be further differentiated from dysplasias. Hyperpigmentation can also indicate dysplastic change if newly diagnosed. This can be seen grossly and confirmed with application of acetic acid with the appearance of acetowhite changes often seen within the hyperpigmented tissue.

5.1.4. Anal Intraepithelial Neoplasia (AIN)

At the junction with the rectum, the anal canal presents a squamo-columnar junction like the cervix. This junctional area is visible and is called the pectinate line, and just like the transformation zone of the cervix it exhibits features of metaplasia. It is particularly vulnerable to the emergence of HPV-related neoplasias. The difficulties encountered in the inspection of the vaginal canal are also present among the folds of the anus and the anal canal. The examination is done by placing the patient in a lateral decubitus and genuflexed, in a lithotomy position if female, or best, bent and tilted forward on a proctologic examination table. After having inspected the perianal area, one uses an anoscope with a water-based lubricant to distend the anal canal. The walls can be cleaned with long swabs called scopettes, which are also used to apply 5% acetic acid. The examination of the anal canal is done while slowly pulling out the anoscope, and abnormal lesions can be selected for biopsy. The use of a colposcope enhances the yield of the examination and is called high-resolution anoscopy. A digital rectal exam is part of the evaluation, especially in the HIV positive patient.

5.1.5. Invasive Carcinoma

The gross appearance of a mass or lesion on the epithelial surface of the lower genital tract organs should prompt immediate biopsy. The keratinizing process leading to such growths may not readily uptake acetic acid and therefore may obviate the need for colposcopic examination if clinical suspicion is already high. Other findings on magnified view of the cervix, vagina, or vulva include friability secondary to necrosis, prominent vascularity from angiogenesis, and irregular contours creating a "sugar-coated" appearance after tumor replacement of normal tissue. The area of most concern should be biopsied by taking a representative sample at the junction of normal and abnormal tissue for direct comparison. Punch or coring type biopsy instruments can be used as well as a pinching type Burke biopsy forceps. Devitalized tissue with erosive changes should be avoided since the ability to evaluate these samples for viable tumor cells may be limited and delay definitive diagnosis.

5.2. Cytology

In general epithelial abnormalities of the cervix are initially recognized by cytology, further evaluated by colposcopy and definitively diagnosed by histology. The indication for referral for colposcopy in nearly all cases is an abnormal cervical cytology.

Cytologic diagnosis in the USA and in many countries is done according to the Bethesda system, proposed in 1988, and revised in 1992 and 2001 (http://www.bethesda2001.cancer.gov). This system has three components: (1) an assessment of the adequacy of the sample for diagnosis; (2) a categorization of the smear (Fig. 5.3); and (3) guidelines for the management of the patient according to the diagnosis. These management guidelines have been revised in 2007 and are freely available at http://www.asccp.org/consensus.shtml.

Table 5.2 summarizes some of the Bethesda system squamous cell abnormalities nomenclature, and how it relates to older systems based on cytology (Papanicolaou) or histology (CIN and dysplasia systems). One of the features of the Bethesda system is a simplification of the previous systems, based on better knowledge of the microscopic appearance and natural history of lesions. Two main categories were thus created, low-grade intraepithelial neoplasia (LSIL) and high-grade intraepithelial neoplasia (HSIL). The Bethesda system also recognizes that some smears show squamous abnormalities that are neither LSIL or HSIL, these atypical squamous cells (ASC) are further divided into ASC of unknown significance (ASC-US) and ASC for which HSIL cannot be excluded (ASC-H).

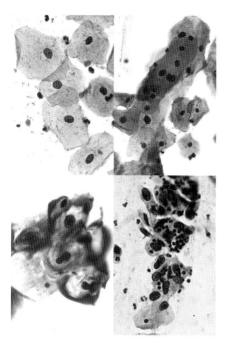

Figure 5.3 *Selected cytologic images of normal superficial and intermediate squamous cells* (top left), *ASC* (top right), *LSIL* (bottom left) *and HSIL* (bottom right)

5.2.1. Atypical Squamous Cells of Undetermined Significance (ASC-US)

It is quite common to detect mildly abnormal squamous cells in cervical smears, which cannot be explained on the basis of any specific inflammatory process and which do not fit into the spectrum of intraepithelial lesions recognized as precursors to squamous carcinoma. This type of abnormality, which has also been referred to in the past as "benign" squamous atypia or borderline dyskaryosis is characterized by a slight to moderate increase in nuclear size and mild nuclear hyperchromasia. It has become clear that this borderline category is truly equivocal in that it correlates with true epithelial abnormality and HPV positivity approximately 50% of the time, compared to samples with unequivocal diagnostic SIL which are more than 90% HPV positive.

5.2.2. Atypical Squamous Cells Cannot Rule Out HSIL (ASC-H)

An important minority of ASC diagnoses is the category of ASC-H. These are smears with cells that are worrisome but felt not to be diagnostic for HSIL. The cells of concern are immature metaplastic cells with a higher N:

Table 5.2 *Different Classification Schemes of Cervical Squamous Cell Neoplasias*

Cytology-based		Histology-based	
Bethesda	**Papanicolaou**	**Cervical intraepithelial neoplasia (CIN) (Richart)**	**Dysplasia (Reagan); World Health Organization**
Normal	Class I	Normal	Normal
ASC-US, ASC-H	Class II		
LSIL		Flat condyloma	Flat condyloma
	Class III	CIN1	Mild
HSIL		CIN2	Moderate
	Class IV	CIN3	Severe
			Carcinoma in situ (CIS)
Invasive cancer	Class V	Invasive cancer	Invasive cancer

Notes: (1) dysplasia is in fact a misnomer. A true dysplasia is a process that affects the embryologic development of a tissue; (2) some pathologists are now favoring grouping condyloma and CIN1 as low-grade CIN (LCIN) and CIN2 and 3 as high-grade CIN (HCIN). *Abbreviations*: ASC-US, atypical squamous cells of undetermined significance; ASC-H, atypical squamous cells, cannot rule out HSIL; LSIL, low-grade squamous intraepithelial lesion; HSIL, high-grade squamous intraepithelial lesion.

C ratio, some degree of hyperchromasia and perhaps mild nuclear contour irregularity compared to benign immature metaplasia.

5.2.3. Squamous Intraepithelial Lesions (SIL)

The degree of severity of an intraepithelial neoplastic process is evaluated on a cytologic sample by a consideration of the morphologic characteristics of the nucleus and cytoplasm of the constituent cells. Cells derived from dysplasia have nuclear areas in the size range of $\sim 3\text{-}4$ times the nuclear area of the reference normal squamous cell nuclei. The nucleus of a normal intermediate squamous cell measures approximately 35 μm^2 and that of a cell derived from an immature squamous metaplasia approximately 50 μm^2. The size varies somewhat with the differentiation of the dysplastic process. Nuclei from HSIL may range from 75 up to 200 μm^2, again depending on the subclass dysplasia.

Other diagnostic features are the chromatin distribution, as well as the staining intensity and pattern. With increasing cytologic grade, there is decreasing cytoplasmic maturity. Mature, well-defined cytoplasm is characteristic of the superficial and intermediate cells of LSILs.

Koilocytotic atypia (KA), the morphologic hallmark of what can be considered human papillomavirus cytopathic effect is most commonly associated with these low-grade lesions. Older synonymous terms including warty atypia, condylomatous atypia or koilocytosis have been used as cytologic diagnoses in cell samples characterized by these features. Microscopically, KA is defined as a cell with an atypical nucleus *and* a clearly defined, sharply delineated perinuclear halo. Hyperchromasia, nuclear enlargement and/or wrinkling of the nuclear envelope or more advanced degenerative changes including a smudging of the chromatin and pyknosis characterize the atypical nuclei. A perinuclear halo alone is not diagnostic.

In contrast HSILs have cells that tend to be derived from areas of less complete differentiation, so-called immature metaplasias. Basaloid, metaplastic appearing cells are closer to the surface with varying but much higher N:C ratios then LSILs and nuclei with all of the above described dysplastic features.

5.3. Histology

The histologic assessment of a cervical biopsy must determine if CIN is present in a sample of epithelium and, if so, the degree of CIN. Both of these decisions may be difficult to make. The former may be difficult because benign and physiological changes may be mistaken for CIN. The latter may be difficult because the features used for interpretation must be evaluated simultaneously in both quantitative and qualitative ways.

CIN is often divided into grades (Table 5.2) as a prognostic aid, implying that the disease evolves through a gradual progression of continuous derangements eventually culminating in a tumor capable of invasion. Although generally true, the correlation between histologic diagnosis and prognosis has uncertainties because in practice one does not wait for cervical cancer to develop.

The defining hallmarks of CIN are its nuclear abnormalities. These include nuclei that are enlarged; pleomorphic (irregular in size and shape) and that often have a wrinkled nuclear membrane. The chromatin is increased in amount (hyperchromasia) and irregularly clumped, often along the inside of the nuclear membrane. Collectively, this constellation of features is described as "nuclear atypia." Often, there is a close correlation between the nuclear abnormality and the amount of differentiation seen. The greater the nuclear abnormality, the lesser is the differentiation observed.

Mitotic activity is the histologic hallmark of cell proliferation. The conceptual distinction between normal and low-grade as well as low-grade versus high-grade CIN has much to do with the frequency, distribution and type of mitotic activity. High-grade CIN has a proliferative phenotype as opposed to low-grade CIN, which while slightly more proliferative in a controlled manner compared to normal is really not characterized by the same kind of viral oncogene driven proliferation as high-grade CIN/HSIL.

The normal squamous epithelium of the cervix has minimal if any mitotic activity, with the mitotic figures being confined to the parabasal layers. In normal or reactive changes, mitotic figures are rare and always restricted to the parabasal cells. In contrast, CIN shows increased numbers of mitoses and they may be present at any level in the epithelium. The frequency of mitoses in the epithelium increases along the continuum from normal epithelium to the most severe forms of CIN. Moreover, the number of mitotic figures in the superficial third of the epithelium increases as the severity of the CIN increases, demonstrating that the vertical position in the epithelium at which mitotic figures are found is a diagnostic indicator useful when contemplating the degree of CIN.

The definition of carcinoma in situ (CIS) requires that the surface epithelium lack all differentiation, so that immature and undifferentiated cells occupy the entire thickness of the epithelium.

In the older nomenclature dysplasias are precursors less severe than CIS. The term mild dysplasia (CIN 1/LSIL) is applied when the proliferating parabasal-like cells are confined to the lower one-third of the epithelium. While many such lesions have koilocytic atypia some do not (Fig. 5.4). Moderate dysplasia (CIN 2) refers to those lesions in which the proliferating cells involve the middle one-third of the epithelium and as these cells involve the upper one-third of the epithelium the dysplasia is considered to be severe (CIN 3). If the entire thickness of the epithelium is replaced by the proliferation the lesion has been termed carcinoma in situ (CIN 3) (Fig. 5.5). The spectrum of CIN 2-3 is thus characterized by cellular proliferation overtaking the epithelium and all are considered HSILs. In the US at least, most CIN2 on biopsy ultimately are proven to be CIN3

Although on histology of CIN2 or less the proliferating cells do not necessarily seem to occupy the full thickness of the epithelium, clearly the entire epithelium is abnormal because cytology, which only samples the surface of the epithelium show abnormalities even in the lowest grades of lesions.

Both cytology and histology suffer equally from less than perfect inter- and intra-observer agreement. This is particularly true for CIN2. It is wrong to consider histology as the gold standard relative to cytology. Both techniques

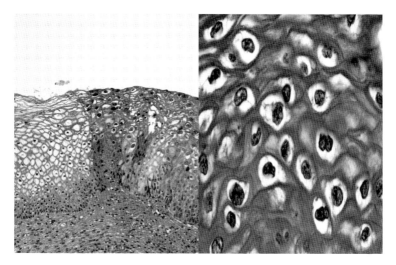

Figure 5.4 On the left one can see the characteristic sharp junction between normal squamous mucosa and LSIL/CIN1. On the right, high magnification demonstrates all the characteristics of koilocytotic atypia associated with productive HPV infection.

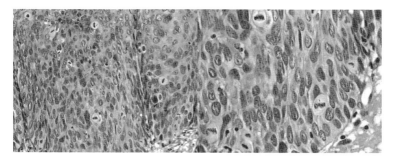

Figure 5.5 On the left a high-grade precancer (CIN3) characterized by full thickness replacement of the epithelium by proliferating cells. Numerous mitotic figures are visible on the right.

have strengths and weaknesses, and it is their combined use that permits better diagnosis and patient management.

5.4. Nucleic Acid Detection Methods

The definitive diagnosis of current human papillomavirus (HPV) infection is made by detection of viral nucleic acids using molecular detection methods. HPV infections are not systemic, but are localized to the epithelium; therefore a direct sample of putatively infected epithelium is required for clinical diagnosis. Most HPV nucleic acid diagnostic tests have been developed specifically for the detection of cervicovaginal HPV infection. While the same tests have been employed in research settings to detect HPV in oral rinses, anal, and penile swabs, the clinical utility of HPV testing from these sites has not been determined. Exfoliated cervical cells can be collected using a variety of sampling devices and collection buffers, however most tests have been developed such that residual material from liquid-based cytology samples can be used for HPV testing.

Some of the commercial HPV nucleic acid detection assays which are compliant with the European Community regulations ("CE-marked') and available in the European Union (EU) are listed in Table 5.3. Only one of these tests, hybrid capture 2 (HC2, Qiagen Corp.), has been approved for clinical use by the US Food and Drug Administration (FDA). It should be noted that while many of these assays have been compared directly to HC2 and demonstrated to have comparable analytic test performance, clinical validity demonstrated through controlled trials is still ongoing in most cases. In general, these tests can be grouped into (1) presence/absence of an internal control for specimen adequacy, (2) those reporting a pooled "high-risk" positive/negative result versus genotype specification, and (3) those targeting viral DNA versus viral mRNA.

5.4.1. Internal Control For Specimen Adequacy

Many tests include a control to ensure the presence of detectable human DNA, which should be present in all clinical samples. This control ensures that the sample was taken and does not contain any material which interferes with the enzymatic processes in the assay. Tests which lack this control risk a higher proportion of false negative samples, since insufficient samples will be recorded as HPV negative.

5.4.2. Pooled High-Risk Detection Vs. Genotyping

HPV type-specific probes in pooled assays are mixed in solution so that a positive result indicates presence or absence of one or more of the high-risk genotypes contained in the pool, but does not allow discrimination of the specific types present. Pooled probes in these assays may also detect low-risk HPV types through probe cross-reaction, leading to false positive test results. HPV type-specific probes in genotyping assays are separated onto a solid membrane surface so that positive signals from each type can be differentiated and results reported on a type-by-type basis.

Table 5.3 Commercially Manufactured Nucleic Acid–Based HPV Assays

HPV diagnostic test	Nucleic acid target
Hybrid Capture 2 (HC2) Qiagen Corp (formerly Digene Diagnostics)	- No internal control for specimen adequacy - Reported as "high-risk positive" or negative - Targets HPV DNA . HPV 16, 18, 31, 33, 35, 39, 45, 51, 52, 56, 58, 59, 68
Roche Amplicor HPV Test Roche Molecular Diagnostics	- Includes internal control for specimen adequacy - Reported as "high-risk positive" or negative - Targets HPV DNA . HPV 16, 18, 31, 33, 35, 39, 45, 51, 52, 56, 58, 59, 68
Third Wave Invader HPV Assay Third Wave Technologies, Inc.	- Includes internal control for specimen adequacy - Reported as "high-risk positive" or negative; also has capacity to subdivide results into 3 groups - Targets HPV DNA . Pool A9 = HPV 16, 31, 33, 35, 52, 58, 67 . Pool A7 = HPV 18, 39, 45, 59, 68, 70 . Pool A5/A6 = HPV 51, 56
GenProbe Aptima HPV test GenProbe, Inc.	- Includes internal control for specimen adequacy - Reported as "high-risk positive," or negative - Targets HPV mRNA . HPV 16, 18, 31, 33, 35, 39, 45, 51, 52, 56, 58, 59, 66, 68
Pretect HPV Proofer NorChip/BioMérieux	- Includes internal control for specimen adequacy - Reported as type-specific result - Targets HPV mRNA . HPV 16, 18, 31, 33, 45
Roche Linear Array HPV Genotyping Test Roche Molecular Diagnostics	- Includes internal control for specimen adequacy - Reported as type-specific result - Targets HPV DNA (37 types) - HPV 6, 11, 16, 18, 26, 31, 33, 35, 39, 40, 42, 45, 51, 52[a], 53, 54, 55, 56, 58, 59, 61, 62, 64, 66, 67, 68, 69, 70, 71, 72, 73, 81, 82, 82v, 83, 84, 89
INNO-LiPA HPV Genotyping *Extra* Innogenetics	- Includes internal control for specimen adequacy - Reported as type-specific result - Targets HPV DNA (28 types) . HPV 6, 11, 16, 18, 26, 31, 33, 35, 39, 40, 43, 44, 45, 51, 52a, 53, 54, 56, 58, 59, 66, 68, 69, 70, 71, 74, 82

[a]HPV 52 status cannot be determined if co-infected with HPV 33, 35, or 58.

5.4.3. Viral DNA Vs. Viral mRNA

Existing nucleic acid-based assays target either the viral DNA or viral mRNA transcripts. The viral oncogenes, E6 and E7 are expressed in higher abundance in the sampled cells from the upper layers of the epithelium of high-grade lesions compared to infected, but cytologically normal samples, whereas viral DNA is present in the upper epithelial layers in women with and without cytological abnormalities. Therefore assays which detect oncogene expression (e.g., E6/E7 mRNA) are more likely to be positive in the present of a high-grade lesion than in a transient infection, potentially increasing the clinical specificity.

5.4.4. Current Status

The evidence to support the value of HPV nucleic acid testing in cervical cancer screening programs is mounting, together with a parallel increase in the number of commercially available HPV assays. Tests should be validated in large clinical trials for the ability to detect high-grade lesions and cancers prior to routine use. At present, HC2 is the only HPV nucleic acid diagnostic test with clear clinical validation though these studies are ongoing for many other assays. Users of HPV nucleic acid diagnostics should be fully cognizant of the layers of validation and standardization required in order to generate reliable test results (Fig. 5.6). While some expert research laboratories can perform HPV nucleic acid detection with a high level of accuracy and reproducibility using in-house protocols and reagents, this practice is strongly discouraged for routine clinical applications.

5.5. Serology

There is currently no commercially available immunoassay for the diagnosis of HPV infections. This is largely because no assay has shown sufficient sensitivity and specificity for clinical use. The antibody response to the different vital proteins during a natural infection is generally weak and inconsistent. The response is strongest and most common against the L1 protein in its native conformation, within a VLP or a capsomere. Many investigators have used VLP of various HPV types in enzyme-linked immunosorbent assay (ELISA) and found antibodies in up to 70% to 80% of patients with an infection with the homologous HPV type. As stated in chapter 1, HPV VLPs generally have a narrow genotype-specificity, in other word genotype = serotype. Nevertheless, some HPV types that are phylogenetically very close, like types 6 and 11 do cross-react. It may take four to six months for antibodies to develop after an infection, and once present antibodies may persist for many years. This is why the main use of serology

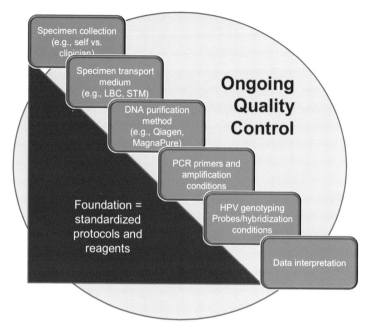

Figure 5.6 *Components of nucleic acid–based HPV assays requiring standardization and quality control. Validated protocols will include recommendations for all components. Changes in any one component from the protocol may decrease validity of test results. Source: From Gravitt et al. 2008.*

is for epidemiologic surveys. Another use for serology has been to ascertain an immune response after vaccination with the current HPV vaccines, which are based on VLPs. The immune response is very strong, and more than hundred fold that observed during a natural infection. Although this response wanes with time, it plateaus at a level still several tenfold higher than after a natural infection. These binding antibodies correlate very well with the neutralization response, which reflects protection against infection. Neutralizing antibodies can be measured indirectly in a competition assay against a known neutralizing monoclonal antibody against the HPV genotype tested. This is the principle of the competitive Luminex Inhibition Assay (cLIA) used in the Gardasil clincal trials. In this assay, VLPs of each vaccine strain are coupled to microspheres and VLP-microsphere complexes are then reacted with pre-/post-vaccination serum samples. Following this, fluorescent labeled HPV genotype-specific neutralizing monoclonal antibodies (MAb) are added and the degree of inhibition of MAb binding is assessed.

Selected References

Web Sites

On colposcopy, high-resolution anoscopy, and cytologyAmerican Society for Colposcopy and Cervical Pathology (ASCCP). Available at: http://www.asccp.org/consensus.shtml.

New York State Department of Health. Available at: http://www.hivguidelines.org.

Articles and Books

Cytology and Histology

Castle PE, Sideri M, Jeronimo J, Solomon D, and Schiffman M. Risk assessment to guide the prevention of cervical cancer. Am J Obstet Gynecol 2007; 197:356.

Castle PE, Stoler MH, Solomon D, Schiffman M. The relationship of community biopsy-diagnosed cervical intraepithelial neoplasia grade 2 to the quality control pathology-reviewed diagnoses: an ALTS report. Am J Clin Pathol 2007; 127:805–815.

Stoler MH, Schiffman M. Interobserver reproducibility of cervical cytologic and histologic interpretations: realistic estimates from the ASCUS-LSIL Triage Study. JAMA 2001; 285:1500–1505.

Stoler M. The impact of human papillomavirus biology on the clinical practice of cervical pathology. Pathol Case Rev 2005; 10:119–127.

Stoler MH. The pathology of cervical neoplasia. In: Rohan T, Shah K, eds. Cervical Cancer: From Etiology to Prevention. Springer, 2004.

Stoler MH. ASC, TBS, and the Power of ALTS. Am J Clin Pathol 2007; 127:489–491.

Nucleic Acid Detection Methods

Gravitt PE, Coutlee F, Iftner T, Sellors J, Quint W, Wheeler C. New technologies in cervical cancer screening. Vaccine 2008; 26 (Suppl 10):K42–K52.

Solomon D, Schiffman M, Tarone R. Comparison of three management strategies for patients with atypical squamous cells of undetermined significance: baseline results from a randomized trial. J Natl Cancer Inst 2001; 93:293–299.

Serology

Stanley M. Immunobiology of HPV and HPV vaccines. Gynecol Oncol 2008; 109: S15–S21.

Dias D, Van Doren J, Schlottmann S, et al. Optimization and validation of a multiplexed luminex assay to quantify antibodies to neutralizing epitopes on human papillomaviruses 6, 11, 16, and 18. Clin Diagn Lab Immunol 2005; 12:959–969.

Screening

Eugene P. Toy
Gynecologic Oncology, Department of Obstetrics
and Gynecology, University of Rochester
School of Medicine and Dentistry, Rochester,
New York, U.S.A.

Mark H. Stoler
Division of Surgical Pathology, Department of
Pathology, University of Virginia Health System,
Charlottesville, Virginia, U.S.A.

Effective screening techniques require detection of a pre-malignant state. The paradigm of cervical cancer screening with use of cervical cytology (Pap smear) is the prime example of such a system. Prior to the advent of cervical cytology, the initial surveys in the United States from the late 1940's reported approximately 33 cases of cervical cancer per 100,000 Caucasian women. In countries where widespread screening is practiced using cervical cytology, this number has decreased to about 4 per 100,000.

Nowadays, cervical cytology is often supplemented by HPV DNA testing.

6.1. Pathophysiology of the Cervix

6.1.1. Pre-menarchal Cervix

The appearance of the cervix early in childhood reflects the germinal tissues which are present at birth. The squamous epithelium which constitutes the vaginal lining is contiguous with the exocervix, which, in this early state of development, is mostly made of the glandular epithelium present from the endocervical canal. The part of the uterine cervix that projects into the vaginal canal, also called *portio*, is made of predominantly glandular tissue whose roughened, red, and friable surface produces mucus, giving the appearance of an *ectropion*.

6.1.2. Adolescent Development

During the process of normal maturation and puberty, the vaginal pH becomes acidic under the influence of ovarian hormones. What was once a prominent glandular *ectropion* now becomes a smooth appearing stratified squamous epithelium that lines the exocervix. This process is called

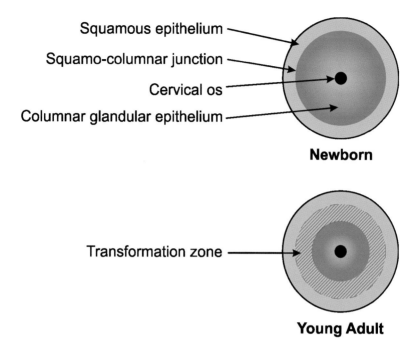

Squamous epithelium
Squamo-columnar junction
Cervical os
Columnar glandular epithelium

Newborn

Transformation zone

Young Adult

Figure 6.1 *Transformation zone of the cervix. The physiologic changes of the cervix that occur during the transition from birth to the early reproductive years are depicted.*

metaplasia. Metaplasia originates at the squamo-columnar junction, which progressively migrates towards the endocervix. This area that has once been glandular and is now squamous epithelium is called the *transformation zone* (Fig. 6.1). This is the area that is at highest risk for developing cervical neoplasia and its sampling for cytology is of paramount importance. Nests of glands retained within the transformation zone often develop inspissated mucous secretions which result in the formation of pinpoint, whitish, pustular lesions called *Nabothian cysts*. These Nabothian cysts may be raised and with surrounding inflammation, and can often be mistaken for a neoplastic process.

6.1.3. Pregnancy

Pregnancy, like puberty, triggers cervical metaplasia. The cervical os becomes both wider and everted, and this exposes to the acidity of the vagina an area that was previously in the endocervix. This creates a new transformation zone. These changes enlarge the region at risk for neoplasia and in need of sampling.

6.1.4. Post-menopausal Changes

In sharp contrast to the changes occurring in pregnancy, the normal aging process and loss of estrogen causes atrophy and shrinkage of both the vaginal and cervical canals. This foreshortening of the cervical tissues moves the transformation zone deeper inside the endocervical canal. Therefore, when collecting cervical cells in a post-menopausal patient one must ensure that the device is able to access the cervical canal and sample the area at greatest risk for neoplasia.

6.2. Screening Techniques

Several precautions need to be taken to obtain the best cervical cytology sample. The collection should not be done during menstruation, and at least for 5 days after the period has stopped. In at least the two days preceding the patient should avoid the following: vaginal intercourse, douching, the use of tampons, as well as the placement of intravaginal devices, medications and contraceptives.

There are two main conventional methods of collecting a sample for cervical cytology. In the conventional method, a special wooden spatula, the Ayre spatula, is positioned in the os and rotated twice, while avoiding excessive mucosal bleeding. The collected material is smeared on a glass slide. To sample the endocervix, one can use a moistened cotton swab, or, better, a cervical brush that is rotated 180°. The collected material is added to the slide, which has to be promptly treated with a cell fixative.

In the liquid-based cytology approach, the sample is collected with a tool called a cervical broom. The device is placed in the cervix and rotated two to four times. The collected material is transferred in a liquid transport medium. There are two commercial systems available, Sure-Path (BD-TriPath Imaging) and Thin-Prep (Hologic Corp). The processing varies according to the system, but the cells end up being spread on a glass slide for examination by the technician or a computer, if appropriate. This liquid-based collection system combined with automated reading overcomes drawbacks such as excess blood or clumps of cells from conventional approach, which can obscure the slide. Another advantage of the liquid based method is that the transport media containing the remaining cells is stored and these cells are available for HPV DNA testing with the commercially available Hybrid Capture II assay. This testing without having to re-sample the patient is called reflex testing, and is done after an equivocally abnormal cytology.

The liquid-based cytology method has enhanced the retrieval of cells thereby decreasing sampling error by fourfold over the traditional method, in which the spatula collection transfers less than 10% of the cells sampled. Cells acquired by cervical brush or broom can approach 95% retrieval.

6.3. Cervical Cancer Screening Recommendations and Triage

In the United States, there are three main sources of cervical cancer screening guidelines. The American Cancer Society (ACS) (http://caonline. amcancersoc.org/cgi/content/short/52/6/342) and the U.S. Preventive Services Task Force (USPSTF) (http://www.ahrq.gov/clinic/uspstf/uspscerv .htm) guidelines are summarized in Table 6.1; the practitioner is advised to use one or the other guidelines and not mix. In addition, the American College of Obstetrics and Gynecology (ACOG) has issued its own guidelines, and the US Centers for Diseases Control (CDC) has added recommendations pertinent to the patient with sexually transmitted diseases (http://www.cdc.gov/std/treatment/).

Table 6.1 Summary of Cervical Cancer Screening Guidelines

When to begin Pap test screening?	
USPSTF, ACS	Approximately 3 yr after a woman begins having sexual intercourse, but no later than age 21 yr
How often?	
USPSTF	Every 3 yr (regardless of the cervical cytology technique used)
ACS	(1) At initiation of screening: Annually with conventional cytology OR Every 2 yr using liquid-based cytology (2) At or after age 30, women who have had 3 consecutive, technically satisfactory normal/negative cytology results may be screened every 2–3 yr Unless (a) they have a history of in utero diethylstilbestrol (DES) exposure (b) are HIV positive (c) are immunocompromised by organ transplantation, chemotherapy, or chronic corticosteroid treatment
When to discontinue screening?	
USPSTF	At age 65 in women who have had normal results previously and who are not otherwise at high-risk for cervical cancer
ACS	At age 70 or older in women with an intact cervix and who have had 3 or more documented, consecutive, technically satisfactory, normal/negative cervical cytology tests, and no abnormal/positive cytology tests within the 10-yr period prior to age 70

Table 6.1 Summary of Cervical Cancer Screening Guidelines (Continued)

When to begin Pap test screening?

Exceptions:
(a) women who have not been previously screened
(b) women for whom information about previous screening is unavailable
(c) women for whom past screening is unlikely
(d) women with a history of: (i) cervical cancer; (ii) in utero exposure to diethylstilbestrol (DES)
(e) women who are immunocompromised (e.g., due to organ transplantation, HIV infection, chemotherapy, or chronic corticosteroid treatment)
(f) women who have tested positive for HPV DNA

Screening after hysterectomy

USPSTF, ACS	Not necessary if (total) hysterectomy was for benign disease

Screening with HPV DNA testing (Hydrid Capture II test for high-risk HPV)

USPSTF	Not recommended
ACS	Can be used with cytology, only at age 30 or older and if both tests are negative they should not be repeated more frequently than every 3 yr

Additional guidelines

ACS	(1) Regular health care visits, including gynecologic care (including pelvic examination) and STD screening and prevention should be done (2) Counseling and education related to HPV infection is critical if HPV DNA testing is done
CDC	(1) Women who have external genital warts do not need to have Pap tests more frequently than women who do not have warts, unless otherwise indicated (2) In HIV-infected women a cervical cytology should be obtained twice in the first year after diagnosis of HIV infection, and if the results are normal, annually thereafter

Web-based Sources:
American Cancer Society (ACS)—http://caonline.amcancersoc.org/cgi/content/short/52/6/342.
U.S. Preventive Services Task Force (USPSTF)—http://www.ahrq.gov/clinic/uspstf/uspscerv.htm.
Centers for Disease Control and Prevention (CDC)—http://www.cdc.gov/std/treatment/.

Cytologic nomenclature is discussed in chapter 5. The one mandated by law in the United Stated is the Bethesda system, which also provides detailed guidelines on how to manage the patient with cervical cytologic abnormalities. These management guidelines have become quite complex and extensive. This section will only discuss the general principles of management, but the reader can access the full recommendations and algorithms, as well as the supporting literature on the web site of the the American Society for Colposcopy and Cervical Pathology (ASCCP) (http://www.asccp.org/consensus.shtml).

6.3.1. Atypical Squamous Cells of Undetermined Significance (ASC-US)

The incidence of ASC-US ranges from about 2% to 4% in most series of screening Pap smears of immunocompetent women. In about 30% of patients with this diagnosis on cervical cytology, there can be subsequent CIN identified. Therefore, the recommendation for these patients with an ASC-US cervical cytology is to undergo reflex HPV DNA testing and determine the presence of high-risk HPV types. If present, the recommendation is to undergo immediate colposcopic evaluation and biopsy. If absent, the patient can be returned to routine surveillance.

6.3.2. Low-Grade Squamous Intraepithelial Lesion (LSIL)

LSIL is a specific cytologic diagnosis based on an increased nuclear to cytoplasmic ratio. When the diagnosis of LSIL is correlated with mild dysplasia or CIN I found on colposcopic biopsy, there is a risk of progression to more severe dysplasia in only about a third of the cases diagnosed. The recommendation for these patients is for continued surveillance with cytology ± colposcopy if indicated by worsening or persistent disease.

6.3.3. High-Grade Squamous Intraepithelial Lesion (HSIL)

The diagnosis of HSIL on cervical cytology screening can have significant implications for triage and subsequent treatment. The range of histologic correlates found on colposcopic biopsy is from moderate to severe dysplasia all the way to carcinoma in situ and invasive carcinoma. The recommendation for these patients is to undergo cervical conization to obtain a larger specimen and to assess for the presence of invasive disease.

6.3.4. Invasive Carcinoma

Frankly invasive carcinoma is infrequently diagnosed on cervical cytology screening. If a gross lesion is present on the cervix, there may be keratinization of the lesion that may give a false negative result to the cervical cytology. Therefore, tissue sampling with biopsy is imperative in cases where the clinician is highly suspicious that a cancer is present.

6.4. Indications for Cervical HPV DNA Testing

The detection of HPV infection is based on the detection of HPV DNA using the commercially available Hybrid Capture II[R] test (Digene Corporation). In this assay, the cells and DNA are denatured. A mix of labeled single-stranded RNA probes for different high-risk HPV types (see chap. 5) is added. These probes bind the complementary single-stranded HPV DNA. The DNA-RNA complexes are then captured by antibodies coating the vial. A photometric measurement gives a semi-quantitative reading of the viral load of the sample. This assay can be performed using the same media from concomitant liquid-based cytologic screening of the cervical cytology.

6.4.1. Adjunct to Cervical Cytology

Reflex HPV DNA testing is recommended in all cases of ASC-US as there can be up to 30% to 50% chance of concomitant dysplasia. If high-risk HPVs are absent, the patient is returned to routine screening cervical cytology with the next smear to be done one year later. If high-risk HPVs are present, the patient is referred to immediate colposcopy with biopsy.

6.4.2. Primary Dual Screening

HPV testing for all patients undergoing Pap smears has been advocated to increase the sensitivity for detecting cervical dysplasia. In the setting of normal cytology, some reports have shown that in patients testing positive for high-risk HPV types, a small percentage will go on to develop HSIL at six month follow-up. The majority of women, however, are found to clear the incident HPV infection. One study of HPV screening of a resource poor population suggested that primary screening with HPV DNA testing, instead of cytology, may provide the greatest benefit for preventing cervical cancer. For now, primary screening with HPV DNA testing in conjunction with cervical cytology is considered beneficial only for women who are over age 30.

6.4.3. Role of Repeat Testing

The large majority of women who test positive for HPV will clear the virus spontaneously. Repeat HPV testing in those that have had negative cytology but positive high-risk HPV DNA will provide reassurance to these women that they are unlikely to contribute to the 4% of women that develop HSIL from this group. In this setting, repeat testing with cervical cytology and HPV DNA is recommended at 12 months. Other unique scenarios supporting repeat HPV DNA testing are in the case of a persistent ASC-US Pap with negative colposcopic evaluation. Finally, those women that have had both negative cytology and negative high-risk HPV DNA on an annual screen may be candidates for combined testing every three years.

6.5. Screening in Special Situations

6.5.1. Pregnancy

Due to the physiologic changes of the cervix during pregnancy noted earlier, the area at risk for development and progression of dysplasia becomes relatively larger. The cervical broom is preferred over the endocervical brush due to the relative risk of bleeding and rupture of membranes. Fortunately, cervical cancer screening in pregnancy allows for the capturing of many previously unscreened women. Pregnancy does not change the management of ASC-US. However, concern for the fetal well-being modifies both triage and subsequent treatment recommendations. The risk of premature uterine contractions along with the increasing blood supply to the uterus and cervix make any colposcopic procedure risky. The safest time is within the second trimester. Endocervical curettage is absolutely contraindicated.

6.5.2. Post-hysterectomy

6.5.2.1. Cervical Cytology Testing

Patients who have had a history of HPV infection and/or dysplasia of the cervix are at most risk for the development of vaginal dysplasia after hysterectomy. The vaginal apex and fornices are the most common location for dyplastic changes to occur in the vagina in the absence of the cervix. Conventional Pap testing can be used to sample the vaginal apex and obtain a representative specimen for the entire vaginal canal. Dysplastic cells of the more distal vagina can also be detected in more proximal locations of the vagina. The results of a simultaneous HPV DNA testing of the vagina and cervix have good correlation. Therefore, in the absence of the cervix, HPV types present in the vagina present the same pathogenic potential as if they had been found in the cervix.

6.5.2.2. Atypical Squamous Cells

In the absence of the cervix, management of atypical cells on a Pap test on vaginal smear is extrapolated from the algorithm established for cervical changes. The mere finding of vaginal atrophy can lead to an ASC-US diagnosis and a short course of vaginal estrogen cream can resolve these changes in several months. Persistent ASC-US on repeat testing or ASC-H should prompt immediate colposcopic evaluation and biopsy.

6.5.2.3. Vaginal Intraepithelial Neoplasia (VAIN)

Guidelines for routine Pap smears of the vagina following hysterectomy for benign indications have been established (Table 6.1). These recommendations do not apply to individuals with a known history of cervical SIL. With regard to these other benign indications, CIN notwithstanding, serial Pap smears are required no more than once every three years.

6.6. Screening for Anal Cancer

The incidence of anal cancer in the HIV population is not only about 10 to 15 times higher than in the normal population, but it is also rising. This and the parallel between the HPV pathogenesis in the cervix and the anus has led to the development of an anal screening approach which is based on anal cytology and if indicated high-resolution anoscopy (HRA), which is the examination of the anal canal with a colposcope. The New York State Department of Health has been the first in September 2007 and only state so far in the United States to have issued guidelines for anal cancer screening (http://www.hivguidelines.org/GuideLine.aspx?pageID=257&guide LineID=22). The target populations are men who have sex with men, any patients with a history of anogenital condylomas, and women with abnormal cervical and/or vulvar histology. There are several reasons why at present this approach has not been more broadly endorsed: (1) the poor to moderate inter- and intra-observer reliability of anal cytology and histology; (2) the complete to partial absence of validation of these screening strategies in the different populations targeted; (3) the limited understanding of the natural evolution of anal HSIL; (4) the near-absence of standardized and validated treatment guidelines; (5) the probably insufficient number of practitioners who can fully manage the diagnosis and treatment of these patients; and most importantly (6) the lack of evidence that this screening has an impact on the prevention of anal cancer.

6.7. New Screening Markers

Several considerations make the development of new screening markers desirable even if perfection far from attainable. The sensitivity of the Pap smear is about 50% to 60% according to the best estimates. Colposcopic biopsy is a poor standard, getting the most severe lesion in only 50% of encounters. Remarkably, biopsy diagnosis is no more reproducible than Pap smear diagnosis. One area of great interest is the use of various molecular markers.

The expression of the E6 and E7 viral oncogenes is thought to be essential for cancer precursor development. E6 and E7 proteins interfere with cell cycle regulation by interacting respectively with the p53 and RB proteins, among the two most important tumor suppressor proteins. Cell proliferation is stimulated and apoptosis is inhibited.

Ki-67 is a marker of cell proliferation that can be detected on biopsies by immunohistochemistry. It may be useful in the problematic biopsy, where the differential diagnosis is between a benign reaction like immature metaplasia or gland regeneration versus a high-grade cancer precursor. $p16^{INK4a}$ is another immunohistochemical marker. This protein is specifically over-expressed when high-risk HPV oncogenes are expressed. About 95% of high-grade cervical lesions and invasive cancers have been shown to express very high levels of $p16^{INK4a}$. Thus on histology, p16 seems reasonably validated for distinguishing high-grade lesions from mimics. The problem is that it is yet to be defined as valid for distinguishing low grade from high grade. Part of the reason for this has to do with biology, the rest with study design in the published studies to date. However large-scale clinical validation trials of p16 are reportedly in the formative stage.

Other immunohistochemical markers that have been investigated include epidermal growth factor, her 2/neu, CEA, MN telomerase, and ProEx C. Some have a biologic rationale, others less so or at least an indirect one. Most of these are very similar to p16 in that they are best correlated with high-grade lesions. However, often the reports on these markers are directly conflicting and the reasons are in the details of study design.

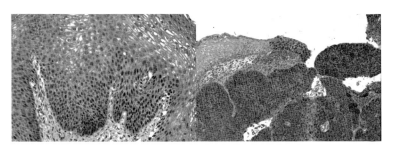

Figure 6.2 Typical p16 immunohistochemical staining patterns (LSIL on left, HSIL on right) marking the nuclei and to a lesser extent cytoplasm of the proliferative cellular compartments activated by the interaction of HPV E7 with the RB protein.

Identifying HSIL with immunohistochemistry is relatively easy. But finding a marker or a small set of easy to implement markers that accurately segregate biopsies into normal versus low grade versus high grade at the 95% level is not quite there yet, although in selected situations they can really help and p16 and Ki-67 are the markers most commonly used as adjuncts in current practice (Fig. 6.2).

Selected References

Web Sites
When to Obtain a Pap Smear

American Cancer Society (ACS). Available at:
    http://caonline.amcancersoc.org/cgi/content/short/52/6/342.
The U.S. Preventive Services Task Force (USPSTF).
    http://www.ahrq.gov/clinic/uspstf/uspscerv.htm.
What to Do with the Results
American Society for Colposcopy and Cervical Pathology (ASCCP). Available at:
    http://www.asccp.org/consensus.shtml.
Care of the HIV Patient
New York State Department of Health. Available at: http://www.hivguidelines.org.

Articles
American College of Obstetricians & Gynecologists. ACOG practice bulletin. Cervical cytology screening. Number 45, August 2003. Int J Gynaecol Obstet 2003; 83:237–247.

Arbyn M, Sasieni P, Meijer CJ, Clavel C, Koliopoulos G, Dillner J. Chapter 9: Clinical applications of HPV testing: a summary of meta-analyses. Vaccine 2006; 24(suppl 3):S78–S89.

Castle PE, Sideri M, Jeronimo J, Solomon D, Schiffman M. Risk assessment to guide the prevention of cervical cancer. Am J Obstet Gynecol 2007; 197:356.

Solomon D, Davey D, Kurman R, Moriarty A, O'Connor D, Prey M, et al. The 2001 Bethesda system: terminology for reporting results of cervical cytology. JAMA 2002; 287:2114–2119.

Stoler MH. Human papillomaviruses and cervical neoplasia: a model for carcinogenesis. Int J Gynecol Pathol 2000; 19:16–28.

Stoler MH, Castle PE, Solomon D, Schiffman M. The expanded use of HPV testing in gynecologic practice per ASCCP-guided management requires the use of well-validated assays. Am J Clin Pathol 2007; 127:1–3.

Stoler M, Castle P, Solomon D, Schiffman M. Expanded use of human papillomavirus testing in gynecologic practice (Correspondence). Am J Clin Pathol 2007; 128:883–890.

Thomison J III, Thomas LK, Shroyer KR. Human papillomavirus: molecular and cytologic/histologic aspects related to cervical intraepithelial neoplasia and carcinoma. Hum Pathol 2008; 39:154–166.

Prevention

William Bonnez
Infectious Diseases Division, Department of
Medicine, University of Rochester School of
Medicine and Dentistry, Rochester, New York,
U.S.A.

Darron R. Brown
Department of Microbiology and Immunology,
Indiana University School of Medicine,
Indianapolis, Indiana, U.S.A.

Cynthia M. Rand
Division of General Pediatrics, Department of
Pediatrics, University of Rochester School of
Medicine and Dentistry, Rochester, New York,
U.S.A.

7.1. Environmental Prevention

There are no specific precautions to control HPV in the environment. HPV are hardy viruses that are relatively resistant to ether, acid, desiccation, and heat. The virus survives to 50°C, but not to 100°C, for 1 hour. Surgical instruments that come in contact with the virus and associated lesions should be sterilized according to standard methods developed for viruses. The presence of papillomavirus DNA in the plume generated by lasers and electrosurgical instruments, and on the walls of the surgical suite, as well the anecdotal reports of hand and nasopharyngeal warts in surgical operators argue for the use of smoke aspiration systems and of protective garments, including goggles, mask, gloves, and gown, when using these instruments for the treatment of HPV-associated lesions. Disposable equipment should be discarded after a single use. Household bleach (5.25% sodium hypochlorite) diluted 1:10 in water is an appropriate disinfectant for contaminated surfaces as well as fomites susceptible to be exchanged, such as sex toys.

7.2. Condoms and Microbicides

It had been difficult to establish whether male condoms are effective in preventing HPV infections and diseases, in large part because in retrospective studies condom usage is difficult to measure reliably. Available

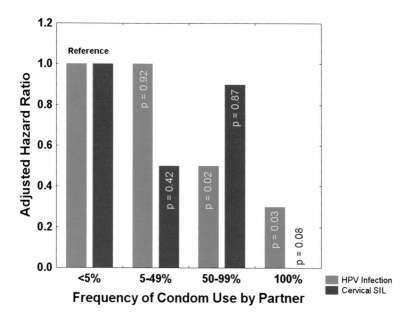

Figure 7.1 Hazard ratios for the association between incident cervical HPV infection or squamous intraepithelial lesion (SIL) and condom use by the male partner. Source: From Winer et al. 2006.

studies indicated a possible beneficiary effect on the transmission of genital warts, CIN2/3, and cervical cancer.

Within the past five years, he work of two groups of investigators has greatly clarified this issue. Rachel Winer and colleagues at the University of Washington examined 82 college-aged women who were virgins three months or less before the beginning of the study. The subjects had gynecologic examinations at study entry and every four months for one year during which cervical and vulvovaginal samples were obtained for cervical cytology and HPV DNA testing. Every two weeks, the subjects recorded their daily sexual activity, including condom use, in a Web-based diary. One hundred percent condom use was associated with a threefold reduction in the risk of cervical, vulvar, and vaginal HPV infection, and frequency of condom use was proportional to that risk (Fig. 7.1). Although not reaching statistical significance, there was a similar decrease of new cervical squamous intraepithelial lesions associated with condom use (Fig. 7.1).

Chris Meijer and his colleagues at VU Medical Center in Amsterdam did a very informative study in which they randomized evenly 125 couples to condom use or not. The women had SIL or CIN at entry. They were examined at entry, three months, and every six months afterward, until they required electrosurgical treatment. The longest follow-up was two years. The women in the group assigned to condom use compared to the non-condom users had a greater clearance of their CIN and cervical HPV DNA by 1.5- and 5.7-folds, respectively. The male partners were also examined, and those who had subclinical flat penile papules, which are known to be associated with HPV, cleared their lesions almost twice as fast if their were assigned to using condoms. The effect of condom use on infection and lesion clearance was consistent with a barrier effect, because it was statistically significant only in the couples who had concordant HPV types.

Although condoms do not offer complete protection against transmission or reinfection by HPV, they have a role in prevention, as long as they are used diligently. They should be recommended when a new sexual relationship is initiated, at least until the risk of exposure to HPV and other sexually transmitted agents can be better assessed. Condom use should also be encouraged while a sexual partner is being treated for an HPV-associated anogenital lesion; however, it is unknown for how long they should be used thereafter.

There are currently no microbicides available that have been clinically proven to be effective reducing HPV transmission. Nonoxynol-9, is a surfactant and spermicide that was once believed on the basis of in vitro testing to be a microbicide as well. Unfortunately, it was later found to be facilitating the transmission of sexually transmitted diseases, including HPV, presumably because the compound causes epithelial disruption. Since then sodium dodecyl sulfate (SDS), an alkyl sulfate surfactant, and carrageenan, a linear sulfated polysaccharide derived from seaweed that is commonly used in the food and cosmetic industry, have been shown in vitro or in animal models to be very effective at preventing, among others agents, HPV and HIV infections. The experience with nonoxynol-9 and the recent failure of carrageenan to prevent HIV transmission in a large randomized clinical trial, emphasize the need for conclusive clinical data before these or any other microbicides can be recommended for HPV prevention.

7.3. Vaccination

7.3.1. Vaccine Preclinical and Early Clinical Development

John W. Kidd, Joseph W. Beard, and Peyton Rous from the Rockefeller Institute showed in 1935 that infection of the domestic rabbit with the Shope papillomavirus derived from the cottontail rabbit, and that causes papillomas and carcinomas, resulted in the production of neutralizing antibodies. Richard

E. Shope, at Yale University, demonstrated the following year that this inoculation was in fact immunizing and protected the domestic rabbit from a second infection. Starting in the 1980s, the wider availability of genetic engineering in *Escherichia coli* encouraged efforts to develop animal papillomavirus vaccines in the cow and in the domestic rabbit model of the cottontail rabbit papillomavirus. These approaches focused on using full or partial fusion proteins of the L1 or L2 genes, or mixtures thereof, as vaccine. The results were variable and not necessarily consistent from one animal species to the other, or within the same species, when comparing the results with bovine papillomaviruses (BPV) 1 or 2, which infect the dermis and epidermis, and BPV-4, which targets the alimentary tract.

In 1944, Hans H. Biberstein described autogenous vaccination for the treatment of genital warts. In this approach, lesions from the patient are used, usually after grinding and filtering, as a therapeutic vaccine to treat the patient's remaining lesions. This approach was later shown to have some success in treating or preventing bovine papillomas and CRPV-induced papillomas. These autogenous vaccines enjoyed some popularity in the cattle industry for whom bovine papillomas of the skin and alimentary tract are an economic burden. This approach received also received renewed favorable attention in the 1970s and early 1980s for the treatment of human genital warts, and even laryngeal warts. The HIV epidemic and the negative results of a randomized, crossover, blinded—unfortunately underpowered—study put an end to this type of vaccination.

The current HPV VLP vaccines came out from a different line of research. In the mid 1980s, many attempts to develop an immunoassay that would detect antibodies against the HPV viral capsid in the blood of patients with genital warts created confusing results. The inability to then grow HPV and produce viral capsids, the paucity of viral particles to extract from genital warts, as well as the rapidly growing multiplicity of HPV types were hurdles to having an appropriate antigen for serology. This forced investigators to use substitutes, denatured or native BPV virions, HPV virions from cutaneous warts, or fusion proteins (i.e., part bacterial and part viral) made in *E. coli* of the full or fragments of the capsid proteins of HPV-6. Altogether, the results from the various the immunoassays, mostly enzyme-linked immunosorbent assays (ELISA) and Western blots, based on these various antigens produced results that were often unimpressive or contradictory. The strongest observation was that about half of plantar warts patients seemed to have antibodies against HPV-1 purified from plantar warts. However, the general relevance of this observation to genital HPV serology was unclear until in the early 1990s the same type of results were obtained with the sera of patients with genital warts or recurrent respiratory papillomatosis using

HPV-11 virions in ELISA. These virions were grown in human skin xenografts implanted in athymic mice, a technique described in 1985 that allowed the production of virions of some of the genital HPV, if fastidiously.

The same animal model was used to show that the serum of a rabbit immunized with intact HPV-11 virions could block the infection of human xenografts when mixed with a challenge inoculum of infectious HPV-11 virions. This demonstration that native, intact HPV-11 virions could induce the formation of neutralizing antibodies was determinant in convincing the investigators, Robert C. Rose, William Bonnez, and Richard C. Reichman at the University of Rochester, that a vaccine might be possible if a capsid antigen could be presented in a native conformation and not be infectious. Different eukaryotic expression systems became available in the late 1980s. In contrast to *E. coli* they had the desirable advantage of not requiring the making of a fusion protein, thus increasing the chance of proper folding of the expressed foreign protein. By 1989 this approach had shown that the capsid protein of several viruses could not only be expressed in a native conformation, but also would spontaneously reassemble to form virus-like particles (VLP) with the same morphology as the native, infectious virions, but without any nucleic acid and thus no infectivity. Whether the making of VLP was a restricted phenomenon, how many capsid proteins were required to make a VLP, and how the antigenic properties of VLP compared to those of homologous infectious virions were largely unknown issues. Efforts were made by Shin-Je Ghim, Richard Schlegel, and A. Bennett Jenson to express HPV-1 L1 protein an SV-40 eukaryotic expression system. However, Jian Zhou and Ian Frazer at the University of Queensland first reported making HPV-16 VLPs in 1991. They stated that L1, the major capsid protein, was alone not sufficient in making VLPs, and that L1 + L2 (minor capsid protein) were required. The structures they called VLPs had neither the size or appearance of what later came to be accepted as correct VLPs, and their immunologic properties were not tested. Indeed, investigators at the National Cancer Institute (NCI), Reinhart Kirnbauer, John Schiller, and Doug Lowy, were unable to replicate that work when they tried using what was understood to be the same strain, the prototype of HPV-16. Rose, Bonnez, and Reichman were able to produce correct HPV-11 VLPs, and later HPV-16, and -18 VLPs, using L1 alone. They also showed that HPV-11 VLP had the same antigenic properties as HPV-11 virions in their ability to detect specific antibodies in the serum of patients with genital warts, but also in inducing neutralizing antibodies. This work was the first solid evidence that there was a close correlation between genotype and serotype. At that time, the NCI investigators were also able to show the synthesis of HPV-16 VLPs with L1 alone, discovering that the prototype strain that they had initially used contained a mutation, not present in the wild-type strains used by the Rochester group, and eventually by them.

The concept of a papillomavirus VLP vaccine was further validated when, in separate experiments, immunization with VLP of canine oral papillomavirus, cottontail rabbit papillomavirus and bovine papillomavirus type 4 of dogs, rabbits, and cows, respectively, gave full or partial protection against challenge by the homologous infectious virus. Passive immunization of naive animals, by transfer of the antibodies of immunized animals, resulted in protection of the animals (dog or rabbit) against challenge infection. These observations established that neutralizing antibodies were responsible and sufficient for protection.

In 1996, the first clinical trials of HPV L1 VLP prophylactic vaccines were started. Investigators at the University of Rochester in collaboration with MedImmune, Inc. worked on HPV-11, while investigators from NCI worked on HPV-16. Both groups showed in dose-ranging studies that these vaccines were strongly immunogenic, that the neutralizing antibodies were generated, and that the vaccines were well tolerated. A cell-mediated immune response was present as evidence by lymphocyte transformation assays, but was not type-specific. The cellular immune response to HPV-16 L1 VLP was later shown more specifically to involve proliferation of CD4+ and CD8+ T cells and in vitro production of T helper 1 (Th1) and Th2 cytokines. The development of the HPV vaccines was then pursued under the control or sponsorship of Merck, which eventually developed Gardasil/Silgard, and GlaxoSmithKline, which made Cervarix. As reflected by the extent of the coverage below, more has been published on Gardasil than on Cervarix.

7.3.2. Gardasil/Silgard

7.3.2.1. Clinical Trials

7.3.2.1.1. Phase I studies In preparation of the clinical studies, African green monkeys were immunized with HPV-11 L1 VLPs. They produced high titer immunoglobulin G (IgG) antibodies that effectively neutralized infectious HPV 11 in the human xenograft athymic mouse system. Antibodies to HPV 11 VLPs were also present in the cervical secretions of the monkeys, but represented only 1% of serum titer.

In order to establish immunogenicity and tolerance, phase I studies were done with different doses of monovalent preparations of HPV-11 and HPV-16 L1 VLPs, administered intramuscularly with a proprietary amorphous aluminum hydrophosphate sulfate adjuvant, at day 0, and months 2 and 6.

The subjects were healthy women with no prior or current serologic and cervical DNA evidence of infection by the HPV type tested. Good neutralizing antibody levels were obtained with doses equal or superior to 50 μg for HPV-11, and 40 μg for HPV-16. This response was still strong three years after vaccination.

In these as in the other studies carried out by Merck, it was not virus neutralization that was directly measured, something that would not be practicably feasible, but rather the ability of the serum from the immunized subject to displace a mouse monoclonal antibody known to bind to the dominant neutralizing epitope of the capsid of a given genotype. A subset of subjects that participated in the phase I evaluation of HPV-16 VLP were followed for the acquisition of HPV-16 cervical infection. None of the vaccinees got infected while 5 cases per 100 person-years at risk did.

Another phase I study was conducted in women regardless of their cervical and HPV serostatus at baseline. This was a dose ranging study of HPV-16 L1 VLP at doses of 0, 10, 20, 40, and 80 μg with three intramuscular injections. Local and systemic reactions were the same in all groups; all subjects received the same dose of adjuvant, amorphous aluminum hydrophosphate sulfate. Those women who were seropositive at baseline had HPV-16 antibody levels 36- to 78-fold higher after immunization. There was a boosting effect of the antibodies developed during a natural infection, because these women had antibody levels after immunization that were 1.1- to 2.4-fold higher than the levels observed in the women who were seronegative at baseline.

The ultimate phase I study was that of the vaccine as a quadrivalent preparation including VLPs from HPV types 6, 11, 16, and 18. This combined a dose escalation protocol on 52 women, followed by a much larger dose-ranging study on 16- to 23-year-old women randomized to received the vaccine with different concentrations of VLP or different concentration of the aluminum adjuvant alone. This study led to the selection of the doses of VLP and adjuvant in the present vaccine, Gardasil. A high immunogenicity sustained for at least three years was documented. Systemic adverse reactions occurred only 13% more often with the current vaccine formulation than with the adjuvant alone, and included headaches (about 40.6%), gastrointestinal disorders (about 24.6%), and fever (about 11%). At the injection site, pain (85.3%), swelling (27.9%), erythema (26.8%), and bruising (4.8%) were the most common manifestations after at least one of the vaccine injections, and occurred up to about 20% more frequently than with the adjuvant alone.

7.3.2.1.2. Phase II studies It was in 2002 that the potential value of the HPV vaccine became established in a striking study by Koutsky et al. HPV-16

VLP (40 µg) or adjuvant alone was administered by intramuscular injections on day 0, and months 2 and 6 to 2392 women aged 16 to 26 years who had had five or less lifetime male sexual partners. The subjects had no history of abnormal Pap smear. They were followed at regular interval with cervical cytology, cervical DNA testing, and serology. Colposcopy was done if indicated. The primary endpoint was the prevention of persistent cervical HPV-16 infection, defined as the detection of HPV DNA at 2 or more consecutive visits. The analysis was done at a 17.4 months of follow-up, after a predetermined number of cases of persistent infection was reached. It was then restricted to women who were HPV-16 serum antibodies and cervical HPV-16 DNA negative at entry. None of the 768 vaccinees and 41 of the 765 placebo recipients had developed a persistent infection, a 100% efficacy [with a 95% confidence interval (CI) of 90–100%]. In a secondary analysis of the control subjects who had developed a persistent infection, 10 of had developed an HPV-16-related CIN. However, there were no differences between the two groups in the rates of CIN not related to HPV-16. The vaccine thus appeared effective at preventing disease as well. As in all the phase I studies that had preceded, the serum anti-HPV-16 levels attained their peak after the third immunization, and slowly declined until the 18th month when they reached a plateau many folds higher than the levels measured after a natural infection. Moreover, the vaccine did not appear to be causing adverse reactions at a rate different from the adjuvant alone. When the results were looked at again after a median follow-up of 48 months, the efficacy of the vaccine was still 94% (95% CI: 88, 98%).

A subset of the subjects enrolled in the dose-ranging study of the immunogenicity of the quadrivalent formulation of the vaccine were evaluated at up to five years for efficacy. These were the subjects who received what was eventually chosen as the Gardasil formulation. The vaccine was 96% effective at preventing a persistent HPV infection by either HPV-16, -11, -16, or -18, and 100% effective at preventing CIN or genital warts related to these genotypes. The subjects who had been followed for at least three years were offered a fourth immunization at month 60, five years after the first immunization. This produced a strong anamnestic antibody response, with levels higher than one month after the third immunization.

In all the studies detailed so far, the most impressive results were observed in vaccine HPV-naive subjects, who were both seronegative and HPV DNA negative. Because these assays are not commercially available, to obtain equivalent results girls should be immunized before they become sexually active and are exposed to genital HPV. Yet, demonstrating efficacy in such young population would take a long time if one were to rely on cervical infection as an endpoint. As preclinical and clinical data had indicated that the presence of neutralizing antibody is a good surrogate of protection, Merck conducted a couple of "bridging" studies in 9- to 15-year-old children to show that the levels of neutralizing antibodies were as high as in 16- to 26-year-olds. It was particularly important that non-inferiority was demonstrated because infections in the older vaccinees had been so rare that no particular protective minimum level of neutralizing antibodies could be defined.

In the first study about 500 each of 10- to 15-year-old boys and girls, about 500 of 16- to 23-year-old women received Gardasil. Depending on the age-class the children had 1.7- to 2.7-folds higher antibody levels than the women, and boys had higher levels than girls. The younger the subject, the higher the antibody level. Fever was more frequent in the children, about 13%, than in the women, 7%. In the second study, about 1800 9- to 15-year-old boys and girls received either Gardasil or the adjuvant alone. By month 18 at least 91.5% of the vaccine recipients were seropositive for a vaccine type. Again, the antibody levels in boys were higher than those of the girls. This sex difference is notable because in natural infections women tend to have a better seroresponse than men. It should be also noted that if the seroconversion rate is not 100%, this is because the assays for the different genotypes in the vaccine do not detect neutralizing antibodies equally well. Local adverse reactions after one or more injections were more common with the vaccine, 75%, than with the placebo, 50%.

7.3.2.1.3. Phase III and IV studies

The prevention of HPV infection by the vaccine was not a satisfactory endpoint if cancer prevention was to be the primary indication. Disease prevention had to be the endpoint. While genital warts could be an acceptable clinical endpoint because they are benign, cancer could not be. For cervical cancer specifically, CIN 2/3 was the best surrogate because it was the immediate precursor, was amenable to secondary prevention by Pap smear and cervical HPV DNA testing if found, was fully treatable, and, most importantly, its detection and removal had been shown to prevent cancer.

Gardasil is made of the L1 VLPs of HPV-6 (20 μg), HPV-11 (40 μg), HPV-16 (40 μg), and HPV-18 (20 μg) made in yeast, mixed with an amorphous aluminum hydrophosphate sulfate proprietary adjuvant (Table 7.1). Four clinical trials (Merck Protocols #005, 007, 013 (FUTURE I), 015 (FUTURE II)) were conducted to demonstrate that Gardasil prevented external genital warts, vulvar and vaginal intraepithelial neoplasias (VIN and VAIN, respectively), CIN and adenocarcinoma in situ (AIS). How the planned analyses were conducted is shown in Table 7.2, while the results

Table 7.1 Summary Information on the Two HPV Vaccines: Gardasil and Cervarix[a]

Name	Gardasil (Silgard in some countries)	Cervarix
Manufacturer	Merck and Co. (distributed by Pasteur-Sanofi in Europe)	GlaxoSmithKline Ltd. (GSK)
Composition	L1 VLPs of HPV-6, -11, -16, and -18, made in *Saccharomyces cerevisiae* (baker's yeast)	L1 VLPs of HPV-16, and -18, made using the *Autographa californica* nuclear polyhedrosis virus (baculovirus) in *Spodoptera frugiperda* (fall army worm) Sf-9 cells and Hi-5 Rix4446 cells derived from another moth larva *Trichoplusia ni* (cabbage looper)
Content	1 dose = 0.5 mL HPV-6 L1 protein: 20 μg HPV-11 L1 protein: 40 μg HPV-16 L1 protein: 40 μg HPV-18 L1 protein: 20 μg Adjuvant: Proprietary amorphous aluminum hydrophosphate sulfate (AAHS), 225 μg Also contains: Sodium chloride L-Histidine Polysorbate 80 Sodium borate Water	1 dose = 0.5 mL HPV-16 L1 protein: 20 μg HPV-18 L1 protein: 20 μg Adjuvant: AS04 = 3-O-desacyl-4'-monophosphoryl lipid A (MPL), 50 μg, adsorbed on hydrated aluminum hydroxide ($Al(OH)_3$), 500 μg Also contains: Sodium chloride Dihydrate sodium monophosphate Water
Preservation	Contains no thimerosal, no other mercury compound, no antibiotic Administer as soon as taken out of the refrigerator (+4°C). Can be left out of the refrigerator at temperatures lower than 25°C for no more than 72 hr	Contains no thimerosal, no other mercury compound, no antibiotic Administer as soon as taken out of the refrigerator (+4°C).

Name	Gardasil (Silgard in some countries)	Cervarix
Route and schedule of administration	Intramuscular injection (deltoid muscle area) at day 0, month 2, and month 6 Notes: -If interrupted, the immunization series should be completed with Gardasil -Dose 2 can be administered at ±1 month, and dose 3 at ±2 months and still yield a satisfactory serologic response	Intramuscular injection (deltoid muscle area) at day 0, month 1, and month 6 Notes: -If interrupted, the immunization series should be completed with Cervarix
Population approved for vaccination (U.S. FDA)	9- to 26-year-old females	Not approved in the United States (in other countries approval based on data collected from 10-to 26-year-old females)
Population recommended for vaccination (U.S. ACIP)	11- to 12-year-old girls 13- to 26-year-old females for catch-up vaccination (some insurers and the Vaccine for Children Fund cover up to age 18 only)	
Approved indications	Prevention of: Cervix: cancer, CIN1-3, AIS Vagina: cancer, VAIN2/3 Vulva: cancer, VIN2/3 External genital warts (condylomata acuminata)	Prevention of: Cervix: cancer and CIN2/3 due to HPV-16/18
Contraindications	Hypersensitivity to any of the vaccine excipients and yeast, including if hypersensitivity was demonstrated after receiving a dose of the vaccine Moderate or severe acute illness	Hypersensitivity to any of the vaccine excipients, including if hypersensitivity was demonstrated after receiving a dose of the vaccine Severe acute febrile illness

(Continued)

Table 7.1 Summary Information on the Two HPV Vaccines: Gardasil and Cervarix^a
(Continued)

Name	Gardasil (Silgard in some countries)	Cervarix
Recommendations for special populations	- Pregnancy: contraindicated - Breastfeeding: not contraindicated, but no data - Hormonal contraceptives: not contraindicated - Immunosuppression: not contraindicated, but immune response may be reduced (no sufficient data) - Abnormal Pap smear: not contraindicated - Positive cervical HPV DNA test: not contraindicated	- Pregnancy: contraindicated - Breastfeeding: not contraindicated, but no data - Hormonal contraceptives: not contraindicated
Administration with other vaccines	Yes Notes: - No interaction demonstrated with hepatitis B immunization - No data yet regarding the administration with the meningococcal vaccine and Tdap (tetanus, diphtheria, and acellular pertussis vaccine), but coadministration is approved by the American Academy of Pediatrics - Each vaccine should be injected at a different site	Yes Note: - No data yet regarding co-administration with other vaccines
Booster immunization Cervical cytology screening Availability	Not recommended at this point Recommendations unchanged by immunization Approved in 103 countries (June 25, 2008)	Not recommended at this point Recommendations unchanged by immunization Approved in 65 countries (June 23, 2008)

^aCheck package insert for approved and current information in the country of use.
Abbreviations: FDA, Food and Drug Administration; ACIP, Advisory Committee on Immunization Practices; CIN, cervical intraepithelial neoplasia; AIS, adenocarcinoma in situ; VAIN, vaginal intraepithelial neoplasia; VIN, vulvar intraepithelial neoplasia.

Table 7.2 Characteristics of the Different Populations in the Planned Analyses of the Phase III Clinical Trials of Gardasil

Criteria	PPE	MITT-2 or Unrestricted Susceptible	MITT-3 or Intention-to-Treat General Population
HPV DNA positive of non-vaccine HPV types at day 1	Included	Included	Included
Seronegative and HPV DNA PCR negative to the relevant vaccine type at day 1	Included	Included	Included
Seropositive and/or HPV DNA PCR positive to the relevant vaccine type at day 1	Excluded	Excluded	Included
HPV DNA PCR positive to the relevant vaccine HPV type during the vaccination phase	Excluded	Included	Included
Pap smear showing ASCUS or higher grade at day 1	Excluded	Included	Included
Protocol violators and recipients of less than 3 doses	Excluded	Included	Included
Case counting	1 month post dose 3	1 month post dose 1	1 month post dose 1

Those who had a normal Pap smear at baseline were considered part of a restricted cohort of MITT-3 called R-MITT-3.
Abbreviations: PPE, per-protocol efficacy; ITT, intention-to-treat; MITT, modified intention-to-treat; ASCUS, atypical squamous cells of undetermined significance.

with up to three years of follow-up are summarized in Table 7.3A. These studies were the basis for the vaccine approval by the U.S. Food and Drug Administration (FDA).

The per-protocol efficacy was to be the benchmark, and the vaccine demonstrated near perfect efficacy against all the clinical endpoints CIN and

Table 7.3A Results of the Main Clinical Trials of Gardasil—Per-Protocol Efficacy (PPE)—Diseases Caused by Vaccine HPV Types

Merck protocol #	Lesion prevented						Caused by HPV			Number of subjects	Vaccine efficacy (95% CI)
	External genital warts	VIN/VAIN		CIN			6/11	16/18	Others		
		I	2/3	I	2/3 & AIS						
005, 007, 013, 015[a]					X			X		17,129	99% (93–100%)
013[b]				X	X		X	X		4,499	100% (94–100%)
007, 013, 015[c]			X		X			X		15,596	100% (72–100%)
013[d]		X					X	X		4,540	100% (49–100%)
013[d]	X						X	X		4,540	100% (92–100%)
019[e]				X	X		X	X		3,819	100% (61–100%)

See Table 7.2 for the definitions of the populations analyzed. In all the studies, the subjects were tightly randomized 1:1 between the vaccine and placebo arms. Except for protocol 019, the subjects were 16- to 26-year-old women, and the results are after up to three years of follow-up. Protocol 019 enrolled 24- to 45-year-old women, and the disease endpoint was assessed by cytology at a mean 1.65 years of follow-up. In that study, the vaccine was 91% effective preventing persistent infection, external genital warts, or CIN caused by HPV-6, -11, -16, or -18.
[a] Joura et al. 2007.
[b] Garland et al. 2007.
[c] Adult 2007.
[d] Koutsky 2007.
[e] Luna et al. 2007.

AIS, VAIN, VIN, and external genital warts. In one of the studies, one woman in the vaccine group was counted as a failure because HPV-16 DNA was detected in one of the histologic specimens. However, this woman had HPV-52 at baseline, as well as in 5 other tissue samples obtained at the time of diagnosis and treatment for CIN3. Twenty seven percent of the enrollees had current or past evidence of at least one vaccine-type HPV infection, with 20%, 6%, 1.2%, and 0.1% having a single, double, triple, and quadruple current or past infection, respectively. Gardasil immunization gave protection against the vaccine-HPV type(s) the women were naive for at baseline, even if they were not naive for the other type(s). In September 2008, the end-of-study results with three to four years of follow-up were reported and remained essentially unchanged. The vaccine efficacy was 98% (95% CI: 93.5, 99.8) for the prevention of CIN2/3 or AIS caused by HPV-16 or -18, 96% (95% CI: 92.3, 98.2) for any CIN or AIS caused by HPV-6, -11, -16, or -18, and 99% (95% CI: 95.2, 99.9) for external genital warts caused by HPV-6, -11, -16, or -18. Efficacy at three to four years of follow-up for VIN2/3 and VaIN2/3 caused by HPV-16 or -18, remained 100%.

As the unrestricted susceptible population analysis demonstrated (MITT-2 analysis in Table 7.2), the vaccine was still very effective against all the endpoint diseases even if the stringency of the analysis was relaxed by including subjects who had an abnormal Pap smear at baseline, did not receive the complete immunization series within one year, or had minor protocol violations (Table 7.3B).

The general population analysis (MIIT-3 in Table 7.2) includes those patients who were not naive to the vaccine-HPV types at entry, and is more reflective of what to expect in clinical practice (Table 7.3C). This cut the efficacy by a quarter to a half depending on the endpoint chosen. This reduction is even more dramatic, a half to four-fifths, if the endpoint was disease caused by *any* HPV types, including non-vaccine genotypes (Table 7.3D). These observations have led to questions about the usefulness of the vaccine. However, these doubts fail to take into consideration several points. The first is that these results were obtained at up to three years of follow-up. With more time one can expect better results as the number of cases accrues faster in the placebo group than in the vaccine group. This supposes of course that the level of neutralizing antibodies will hold up for more than three years, but at five-year follow-up this assumption appears to be correct (see previous section).

Second, the results shown vary substantially according to the geographic area reflecting the local prevalent HPV type distribution. They are indeed twofold better in North America than in Asia. This is not to say that the vaccine has no value in Asia, because, and this is the third point, high-risk

Table 7.3B Results of the Main Clinical Trials of Gardasil—Unrestricted Susceptible Population (MITT-2)—Diseases Caused by Vaccine HPV Types

Merck protocol #	Lesion prevented					Caused by HPV			Number of subjects	Vaccine efficacy (95% CI)
	External genital warts	VIN/VAIN		CIN		6/11	16/18	Others		
		1	2/3	1	2/3 & AIS					
005, 007, 013, 015					X		X		19,466	98% (93–100%)
013				X	X	X	X		4,951	98% (92–100%)
007, 013, 015			X				X		17,531	97% (79–100%)
013		X				X	X		5,351	82% (16–98%)
013	X					X	X		5,351	96% (86–99%)

Notes: See Table 7.2 for the definitions of the populations analyzed. Sources and additional information are given in Table 7.3A.

Table 7.3C   Results of the Main Clinical Trials of Gardasil—Intention-to-Treat Population (MITT-3)—Diseases Caused by Vaccine HPV Types

Merck protocol #	Lesion prevented					Caused by HPV			Number of subjects	Vaccine efficacy (95% CI)
	External genital warts	VIN/VAIN		CIN		6/11	16/18	Others		
		I	2/3	I	2/3 & AIS					
005, 007, 013, 015					X		X		20,583	44% (31–55%)
013				X	X	X	X		5,455	55% (40–66%)
007, 013, 015			X				X		18,174	71% (37–88%)
013		X				X	X		5,455	63% (<0–88%)
013	X					X	X		5,455	76% (61–86%)

Notes: See Table 7.2 for the definitions of the populations analyzed. Sources and additional information are given in Table 7.3A.

Table 7.3D Results of the Main Clinical Trials of Gardasil—Intention-to-Treat Population (MITT-3)—Diseases Caused by Any HPV Types

Merck protocol #	Lesion prevented					Caused by HPV			Number of Subjects	Vaccine efficacy (95% CI)
	External genital warts	VIN/VAIN		CIN		6/11	16/18	Others		
		I	2/3	I	2/3 & AIS					
005, 007, 013, 015					X		X	X	20,583	18% (7–29%)
013				X	X	X	X	X	5,455	20% (8–31%)
007, 013, 015			X				X	X	18,174	49% (18–69%)
013		X				X	X	X	5,455	18% (<0–46%)
013	X					X	X	X	5,455	51% (32–65%)

Notes: See Table 7.2 for the definitions of the populations analyzed. Sources and additional information are given in Table 7.3A.

HPV types are not equally oncogenic. HPV-16 and -18 are the most oncogenic HPV types, but they are also relatively less prevalent in CIN2/3 lesions, and even more so in CIN1, than they are in cervical cancers. Therefore, the impact of the vaccine is expected to be greater on the prevention of cervical cancer than of CIN2/3, and even greater than on the prevention of CIN1. Nevertheless, is spite of these limitations, in the clinical trials Gardasil cut the rate of HSIL by half.

Finally, vaccination has a niche to fill that even cervical cytology cannot. In the United States, 50% and 10% of cervical cancers occur in women who have either never been screened, or not screened in the past five years, respectively. Assuming that the factors leading to this inadequate screening were to remain unchanged, as they mostly have to do with poverty, they would not be significant barriers to childhood immunization, which for the poor is entirely supported by the Vaccine for Children Fund. In addition, vaccination requires 6 months of compliance, whereas for cervical cytology screening it is approximately 50 years. Furthermore, HPV vaccination also provides protection against HPV-associated diseases for which screening does not exist, like in the vulva and vagina.

A Phase II study of Cervarix (see below) had shown that the protective effect of HPV vaccination was not strictly limited to the genotypes included in the vaccine (Table 7.4). Immunization with types 16 and 18 offered also partial protection against new (incident) infections caused by types 31, a relative of type 16, and type 45, a relative of type 18. The same cross-protection was also seen with Gardasil (Table 7.4). The Gardasil studies were further analyzed for a protective effect against incident diseases, not just infections, caused by non-vaccine HPV. In subjects naive to all 14 HPV types (6, 11, 16, 18, 31, 33, 35, 39, 45, 51, 52, 56, 58, 59) tested at entry, Gardasil was 59% effective at giving protection against CIN2/3 and adenocarcinoma in situ (AIS) caused by HPV types 31 and/or 45. This efficacy was still 43% if one included subjects naive to at least one of the 14 HPV types tested. These results have led to the addition by the European Medicines Agency (EMEA) of cross-protection against HPV-31/45 CIN2/3 and AIS in the Gardasil indications.

Merck also conducted a study of Gardasil in 3819 women aged 24 to 45 years who had no history of genital warts or of cervical LEEP or hysterectomy, and were evenly randomized to vaccine or placebo. At 2.2-year follow-up, according to the per-protocol analysis using HPV6/11/16/18-related any CIN or external genital warts as endpoint, the efficacy was 92% (1 count in the vaccine group and 13 in the placebo group). There was no obvious effect of age on the efficacy rate. No indication has been granted yet for immunization in this older age group.

Table 7.4 *Cross-Protection Efficacy Results (MITT-2-Population)*

Persistent infection (for 5 months or more)	Gardasil Phase II/III dataset (Merck)		Cervarix PATRICIA (GSK)	
	% Reduction	95% CI	% Reduction	97.9% CI
HPV-31/33/45/52/58 persistent infection	18.9	5.9, 30.2	ND	ND
HPV-31	47.4	27.0, 62.5	36.1	0.5, 59.5
HPV-33	31.3	−12.9, 58.7	36.5	−9.9, 64.0
HPV-45	22.2	−21.6, 50.6	59.9	2.6, 85.2
HPV-52	5.3	−26.3, 29.0	31.6	3.5, 51.9
HPV-58	12.5	−25.7, 39.2	−31.4	−132.1, 24.7
Any non-vaccine oncogenic HPV type[a]	22.8	9.8, 33.9	9.0	−5.1, 21.2
Any oncogenic HPV type[b]	42.7	33.7, 50.5	21.9	10.7, 31.7

[a]For Merck: 31, 33, 35, 45, 52, 58, 59; for GSK: 31, 33, 35, 39, 45, 51, 52, 56, 58, 59, 66, 68.
[b]For Merck: 16, 18, 31, 33, 35, 45, 52, 58, 59; for GSK: 16, 18, 31, 33, 35, 39, 45, 51, 52, 56, 58, 59, 66, 68.

In a review of over 12,000 subjects aged 9 to 26 years who had received either vaccine or placebo, it was observed that the neutralizing serological response was inversely proportional to the age at immunization. Furthermore, immunization of someone with pre-existing antibodies led to higher response than in somebody who did not have baseline antibodies. The same review failed to detect any effect on immunogenicity of race or ethnicity, region of residence, lactation status, hormonal contraceptive usage, smoking status, Pap smear status, or use of immunosuppressant or anti-inflammatory drugs. These latter findings are reassuring given that an in vitro and animal study had signaled a potential inhibitory effect of cyclooxygenase(cox)–2 inhibitors on the immune response to HPV-16 VLPs.

An apparent increase of non-vaccine HPV-related CIN2/3 or AIS in the vaccinees relative to the placebo recipients has mystified some reviewers. This effect is due to the fact that case counting is done whenever a vaccine HPV-related lesion is observed. In the placebo group, any lesion related to a non-vaccine type would not be counted if it is detected in a patient *after* a vaccine HPV-related lesion has already been counted. Since in the vaccine group those vaccine HPV-related lesions almost never occur, all the non-vaccine HPV-related lesions can be counted, creating a spurious "replacement" effect of vaccine HPV-related lesions by non-vaccine HPV-related ones.

The current package insert of Gardasil states that the vaccine is not effective in preventing against lesions due to an HPV type for which the subject has evidence of prior or current infection. However, longer follow-up to 44 months of the subjects described in Table 7.3B and belonging to protocols # 005, 013, and 015 has allowed an accrual of more cases. A MITT-2 analysis (see Table 7.2 for definition) of these data, presented to the U.S. Centers for Diseases Control and Prevention (CDC) Advisory Committee on Immunization Practices (ACIP) in February 2008, showed that the vaccine efficacy was 100% (95% CI: 29, 100) against HPV-6, -11, -16, or -18-related CIN in the subjects who were at baseline were seropositive but HPV DNA negative for the relevant type. Based on trends so far reported, it is not excluded that the vaccine may also show some efficacy in the seronegative, but HPV DNA positive subjects, meaning that the vaccine could help reduce the transition rate from infection to disease.

The results of a study evaluating the efficacy of Gardasil in males for the prevention of external genital wart were reported in November 2008. 4065 heterosexual men (aged 16 to 23 years) and men having sex with men (about 600, aged 16 to 26 years) were enrolled to received Gardasil or placebo. One month after the vaccination phase they were followed every 6 months, and had samplings of the penis, scrotum, and anus (MSM only) for HPV DNA. Biopsy-confirmed external genital warts, as well as penile, perineal, and perianal intraepithelial neoplasia or cancer were the clinical endpoints. After a mean duration of follow-up of 29 months, the vaccine was 90.4% (95% CI: 69.2, 98.1) effective (per-protocol evaluation) at preventing any vaccine HPV-related external lesion (3 cases in the vaccine group and 31 cases in the placebo group). Vaccine efficacy was 89.4% (95% CI, 65.5, 97.9) against external genital warts and 100% (95% CI, <0, 100) against penile, perineal, and perianal intrapithelial neoplasias (3 cases in the placebo group). There were no cases of cancer in either group.

The Nordic countries (Denmark, Sweden, Norway, and Finland) will be the site of the phase IV studies of HPV vaccination for both Gardasil and Cervarix. Each of these countries has a mass-screening program for cervical cancer with a central registry that will allow to assess the duration of vaccine effectiveness, the impact of vaccination on rates of cervical cancer, and long-term complications. The baseline HPV status, disease burden in the population has been assessed in the three years prior to the introduction of the vaccine. Since the introduction of the vaccine, the disease burden is beingmonitored annually for 5 years, and at the end of that period a survey will assess the HPV status of the population. Almost 5500 Nordic females were enrolled into Protocol 015 and are to be followed through this registry. Protocol 018 is an adolescent study that enrolled 9- to 18-year-old adolescents. It is extended to collect immunogenicity data at 10 years, with an interim analysis at 5.5 years after dose 3.

7.3.2.2. The Vaccine

Table 7.1 summarizes the practical information about the vaccine. Patient education is an integral part of vaccine administration. The following key information need to be provided, modified according to the approved indications specific for the country of use (please consult the package insert): (1) immunization does not change the need or frequency of cervical cancer screening; (2) because the vaccine is not protective against (at least most of) the HPV types not in the vaccine, it is still possible to develop vulvar, vaginal, or cervical HPV-related diseases or abnormalities; (3) the vaccine does not protect (at least as well) against vaccine or non-vaccine genital HPV types if the woman has been exposed to them prior to immunization; (4) not all genital diseases are caused by HPV; (5) although probably uncommon the vaccine may not give protection to all vaccine recipients; and (6) there is no evidence that the vaccine has any therapeutic effect against the diseases it prevents. There is evidence that the vaccine is effective in women aged 27 to 45 years and in males aged 16 to 26 years, but this is not an approved indication at present.

The duration of the vaccine protection is of at least five years for the main endpoint of CIN2/3, AIS, and external genital warts. Because protection is felt to be solely dependent on the neutralizing activity of the serum after immunization, the decay of the serum neutralizing antibody activity based on the data collected so far can be modeled to try to estimate how long the immunity will last. This approach suggests that it will take at least 12 years for the vaccine HPV antibody levels to reach those created by a natural infection. It is therefore impossible to say at this point if and when a booster immunization will be needed.

7.3.2.3. Adverse Events

7.3.2.3.1. Observed during the clinical trials   Table 7.5 summarizes the local adverse reactions observed during the clinical trials of Gardasil. Pain at the

Table 7.5 *Injection Site Adverse Reactions with Gardasil, the Adjuvant Alone, and Normal Saline Placebo*

	Gardasil n = 5088	AAHS[a] control n = 3470	Normal saline placebo n = 320
Pain	83.9%	75.4%	48.6%
Swelling	25.4%	15.8%	7.3%
Erythema	24.7%	18.4%	12.1%
Pruritus	3.1%	2.8%	0.6%

[a]Amorphous aluminum hydrophosphate sulfate (AAHS) adjuvant.
Source: Barr and Sings (2008).

injection site was the most common one, swelling and erythema were less than a third less common. Few subjects (0.1%) discontinued due to adverse experiences. A total of 24,274 subjects (Gardasil 13,686, adjuvant alone 11,004, normal saline placebo 584) aged 9 through 45 years for the females, and 9 through 15 years for the males, were immunized; 237 (0.97%) reported a serious adverse event. Only 0.05% of the serious reactions were judged to be vaccine related. The most frequently reported adverse events were headaches, gastroenteritis, appendicitis, pelvic inflammatory diseases, urinary tract infection, pneumonia, pyelonephritis, pulmonary embolism, bronchospasm, asthma, injection site pain, injection site movement impairment.

Twenty-four deaths occurred. All were consistent with causes of deaths anticipated in a health adolescent and adult population. They included motor vehicle accidents, overdose/suicide, pulmonary embolism/deep venous vein thrombosis, sepsis, pancreatic cancer, arrhythmia, asphyxia, pulmonary tuberculosis, hyperthyroidism, postoperative pulmonary embolism and acute renal failure, systemic lupus erythematosus, acute lymphocytic leukemia, medulloblastoma.

Although subjects were supposed to avoid pregnancy, 3620 of the 16- to 45-year-old subjects did report at least one pregnancy (1796 with Gardasil, 1824 with the adjuvant or saline). Adverse outcome (defined as the combined number of spontaneous abortions, late fetal death, or congenital anomalies for all the pregnant women whose outcome was known, excluding elective terminations) were 23.3% (423/1812) for Gardasil, and 24.1% (438/1820) for the adjuvant or saline recipients. Serious adverse reactions were observed in 54 (rate of 3.0%) Gardasil vaccinees, and 63 (rate of 3.5%) adjuvant or saline recipients. Congenital anomalies occurred in 40 of the pregnancies of Gardasil vaccinees, and 53 of the pregnancies of the adjuvant or saline recipients. When the cases were analyzed according to whether the vaccination occurred within 30 days of conception or 30 days or greater, the ratio of Gardasil versus adjuvant or saline cases was 5:1 and 35:29, respectively.

7.3.2.3.2. Observed after approval   Some of the information available comes from the Vaccine Adverse Event Reporting System (VAERS) managed by the U.S. FDA and CDC. Anybody, not necessarily a physician or a patient can report to VAERS. Dizziness (13%), syncope (10%), injection site pain (19%), nausea (9%), pain (7%), and rash (7%) were among the seven most frequently reported symptoms. Syncope with sometimes a fall resulting in injury led the ACIP to recommend the observation of the patient for 15 minutes after administration of the vaccine.

As of April 30, 2008, 12 million doses of Gardasil had been distributed in the United States and 7802 reports had be made to VAERS. Among those were 31 reports of Guillain-Barré syndrome, 10 of which were confirmed; 5 of them occurred with the concurrent administration of the meningococcal vaccine (Menactra). Of the 21 unconfirmed cases, 7 did not meet the case definition, 1 had symptoms before vaccination, 4 were unconfirmed, and 9 were awaiting additional follow-up. Fifteen deaths were reported. Ten of the cases had enough information. It was concluded that no causal association could be made with the administration of Gardasil. CDC supports since 2001 the Clinical Immunization Safety Assessment (CISA) network, which regroups six academic centers with vaccine safety expertise. Two of these centers, Johns Hopkins University and Boston Medical Center, have respectively reviewed the cases of transverse myelitis and Guillain Barré syndrome that have been reported to VAERS from the time of Gardasil licensure up to August 2008. By that time almost 20 million doses had been dispensed. Two cases of transverse myelitis, and 9 cases of Guillain Barré syndrome (4 had also received the meningococcal vaccine Menacta) occurred within 4 to 42 days after vaccination. The evidence to establish a causal link was deemed insufficient. This study also showed that most cases of Guillain Barré syndrome did not meet the case definition.

A database like VAERS relies on voluntary reporting, and this can lead to an under- or overestimation of the the adverse events associated with HPV vaccination. This is demonstrated by a study done in a cohort of adolescent and young women enroled in the Northern California Kaiser Permanente Medical Care Program, which asked based on the rates of emergency consultations, hospitalizations, and outpatient consultations in 2005 (before the introduction of Gardasil) what would be the rates of immune-mediated adverse events that would occur by chance in close temporal association with HPV vaccination. Thyroiditis was much more common than Guillain-Barré syndrome or multiple sclerosis, yet it tends to be under-reported, presumably because unlike the two other conditions it does not have the reputation of being a possible complication from vaccination.

In order to have a more accurate assessment of the adverse events that are associated with HPV vaccination, CDC has several other surveillance studies in place.

The HPV Vaccine Impact Monitoring Project (HPVIMP) is monitoring vaccine history in a population of women with CIN2/3 or AIS at participating sites in four different states. The STD Surveillance Network (SSuN) is developing tools to assess the descriptive epidemiology, HPV vaccine use, and treatment outcome in patients with genital warts attending sexually transmitted diseases (STD) clinics.

The Vaccine Safety Database (VSD), established in 1990, is a collaboration between CDC and 8 managed care organizations (8.8 million members or 3% of the US population). It conducted from August 20, 2006 through July 20, 2008 a rapid cyle analysis (RCA) at 7 VSD organizations to identify associations between Gardasil immunization and a pre-specified list of adverse outcomes (including Guillain Barré syndrome, seizures, syncopes, strokes, and venous thromboembolism) in females aged 9–26 years. A preliminary analysis reported to the ACIP on about 378,000 doses administered failed to find any statistically significant risk for any of the pre-specified conditions. There was also no major significant increase in the number of cases of anaphylaxis associated with the deployment of the vaccine.

7.3.3. Cervarix

7.3.3.1 Clinical Trials

7.3.3.1.1. Phase I studies Cervarix is a bivalent vaccine that is made of the L1 VLP of HPV-16 (20 µg) and HPV-18 (20 µg) made in a baculovirus (an insect virus) expression system. These VLPs are mixed with an AS04 adjuvant. This adjuvant is made of 500 µg of aluminum hydroxide and 50 µg of 3-*O*-deacyl-4′-monophosphoryl lipid A (MPL). MPL is a detoxified lipid A derived from the lipopolysaccharide of *Salmonella minnesota* R595.

In preclinical and clinical phase I studies this vaccine was given intra-muscularly at day 0, and months 1 and 6 to mice, monkeys, and human volunteers. Controls were given the same VLP preparation, except for the adjuvant which was aluminum hydroxide without MPL. Antibody titers to HPV-16 and -18 VLPs were 1.6- to 8.5-fold higher with the AS04 adjuvant than with the aluminum hydroxide alone, and antibody persisted for at least 3.5 months.

7.3.3.1.2. Phase II studies   The immunogenicity, tolerance, and efficacy of Cervarix was demonstrated in a study that included 1113 females ages 15 to 25 years who were randomized to receiving either Cervarix or the adjuvant alone by intramuscular injection at month 0, 1, and 6. The primary endpoint was the prevention of HPV-16 or -18 cervical infection in women who were seronegative and HPV DNA negative for these two viruses at entry, and who were as well cytologically negative. A secondary endpoint was the prevention of persistent HPV-16 or -18 infection, and another endpoint was the prevention of cytologic or histologic atypical squamous cells of unknown significance (ASCUS), CIN, or cancer. Seroconversion after vaccination occurred in 98% or more of the subjects, up to 5.5 years. As with Gardasil, the titers were higher that those observed after a natural infection.

At up to 18 months of follow-up, in the cohort followed according to protocol (366 vaccine an 355 placebo recipients), the vaccine efficacy was 91.6% (95% CI: 64.5, 98.0) for incident HPV-16 or -18 infections, 100% (95% CI: 47,100) for persistent infections, and 92.9% (95% CI: 70, 98.3) for cytologic ASCUS or higher. The analysis was repeated at 4.5 years of follow-up, still giving excellent results of 96.9% (95% CI: 81.3, 99.9), 94.3% (95% CI: 63.2, 99.9), and 95.7% (95% CI: 83.5, 99.5), respectively. Using CIN2/3 by cytology or histology caused by HPV-16 or -18 as the endpoint, the efficacy was 100% (95% CI: -7.7, 100). Cervarix was also shown to give some cross-protection against HPV-31 (54.5% efficacy) and HPV-45 (94.2% efficacy) infections (Table 7.4).

The immunogenicity of Cervarix was studied in a group of 10- to 25-year-old females. Seroconversion was 100% for binding antibodies to HPV-16 and -18, which were subsequently shown to correlate very well with neutralizing antibodies, but are easier to measure and a more sensitive measurement of seroconversion. In that study (Protocol HPV-012), the 10- to 14-year-old females had antibody titers about twofold higher than those of the 15- to 25-year-old females, thus repeating an observation on the effect of age at immunization also made with Gardasil. In Protocol HPV-014, Cervarix immunogenicity was evaluated in 26- to 55-year-old women. The antibody titers were slightly lower than in 15- to 25-year-old females, but still well above those developed after a natural infection.

7.3.3.1.3. Phase III and IV studies   As with Gardasil, in order to obtain regulatory approval, Cervarix evaluation had to show efficacy preventing HPV high-grade CIN. This phase III study (protocol HPV-008, also known

Table 7.6 *Comparison of the Design of Pivotal Efficacy Trials for Gardasil (Merck) and Cervarix (GSK) Vaccines*

Parameter	Gardasil Phase II/ III dataset (Merck)	Cervarix PATRICIA (GSK)
Sample size	20,541	18,644
Key inclusion criteria		
Age range	16–26	15–25
Number of lifetime sex partners at day 1	0–4	0–6
Key exclusion criteria		
Visible genital warts	Yes	No
Missing cytology	No	Yes
HSIL Pap test at day 1	No	Yes
Comparator	Adjuvant (amorphous hydrophosphate sulfate) placebo	Hepatitis A vaccine with AS04 adjuvant
Visit schedule		
Screening cytology	6- to 12-month intervals	12-month intervals
Colposcopy referral	Protocol-dependent	Aggressive
Cervicovaginal sampling	6- to 12-month intervals	6-month intervals
Primary endpoint	HPV-16/18-related CIN2/3 or AIS	HPV-16/18-related CIN2/3 or AIS
Main analysis population	MITT-2	PPE

Abbreviations: PPE, per-protocol evaluation; MITT, modified intention-to-treat population. See Table 7.2 for definitions.

as PATRICIA) has been reported only in an interim form. Tables 7.6–7.8, summarize some of the designs and results of this study, and compare them to the phase III studies of Gardasil. PATRICIA enrolled 18,644 women 15 to 25 years of age, regardless of their HPV DNA or cytology status (however, women with high-grade cytology were excluded from the interim analysis). They were randomized to intramuscular immunization at day 0, months 1 and 6 with either Cervarix or GSK hepatitis A virus (HAV) vaccine, which served as a control because it contains the same adjuvant as Cervarix. The primary endpoint was histologically proven CIN2 or higher (CIN2+) associated with HPV-16 or -18. Cases were counted after the first

Table 7.7 Comparison of Baseline Characteristics Between the Trials for Gardasil (Merck) and Cervarix (GSK) Vaccine

Parameter	Gardasil Phase II/ III dataset (Merck)	Cervarix PATRICIA (GSK)
Mean age (yr)	20	20
Region of origin		
Asia Pacific	4%	34%
Europe	44%	35%
Latin America	27%	15%
North America	25%	16%
Ethnicity		
Asian	4%	31%
Black	5%	4%
Hispanic	12%	7%
White	71%	87%
Other	9%	2%
Day 1 HPV DNA status		
HPV-16 naïve	83%	81%
HPV-16 PCR positive	9%	5%
HPV-18 naïve	93%	87%
HPV-18 PCR positive	4%	2%
Day 1 cytology		
Negative	88%	90%
ASC-US/LSIL	11%	9%
HSIL/ASC-H/AGC	0.9%	0.5%

Abbreviations: HSIL, high-grade squamous intraepithelial lesion; ASC, atypical squamous cell; ASC-US, ASC of undetermined significance; ASC-H, ASC, cannot rule out HSIL; AGC, atypical glandular cell.

vaccine dose. The interim analysis was to be triggered when the number of cases of CIN2+ in the whole study was to reach 23.

Table 7.8 shows some of the results done in the subjects who were seronegative and HPV DNA negative at entry for the HPV type evaluated. When the analysis included subjects who either seropositive or seronegative to HPV-16 or -18, the vaccine efficacy was 91.6% (97.9% CI: 60.2, 99.4). There were an unexpected high number of multiple infections (61%) among the 23 cases. This led to a post hoc algorithm of case counting to take into account the pattern of HPV types present in the infections prior to the histologic diagnosis. In that analysis, the vaccine efficacy was 100% (97.9% CI: 74.2, 100).

Table 7.8 Main Efficacy Results for Gardasil and Cervarix

Endpoint	Gardasil Phase II/III dataset (Merck)		Cervarix PATRICIA (GSK)	
	% Reduction	95% CI	% Reduction	97.9% CI
HPV-16/18-related CIN2/3 or AIS	97.5	92.6, 99.5	90.4	53.4, 99.3
HPV-16	97.1[a]	91.3, 99.4	93.3	47.0, 99.9
HPV-18	100.0	84.1, 100.0	83.3	−78.8, 99.9
HPV-16/18-related CIN or AIS	ND	ND	89.2	59.4, 98.5
HPV-16	95.0[b]	89.5, 98.0	88.9	44.6, 99.2
HPV-18	94.5[b]	83.2, 98.9	90.9	22.1, 99.9
Persistent HPV-16/18 infection (for 5 months or more)	92.9[c]	88.4, 97.0	80.4	70.4, 87.4
HPV-16	93.9	88.9, 97.0	84.1	73.5, 91.1
HPV-18	90.8	80.0, 96.4	74.0	49.1, 98.8
Persistent HPV-16/18 infection (for 10 months or more)	ND	ND	75.9	47.7, 90.2
HPV-16	ND	ND	79.9	48.3, 93.8
HPV-18	ND	ND	66.2	−32.6, 94.0

[a]Protocols 005, 007, 013 (FUTURE I), 015 (FUTURE II).
[b]Protocols 007, 013, 015.
[c]Protocol 012.

This study, like the phase II study revealed a cross-protective effect of the vaccine against HPV-31 and HPV-45 infections persistent for six months or more (Table 7.4).

The Nordic countries, as with Gardasil, are the site chosen to establish the effectiveness of Cervarix against cervical cancer.

7.3.3.2. The Vaccine

Table 7.1 summarizes the information about the vaccine. The education of the patient or of her guardian is integral to the administration of the vaccine. The content of the information to convey has already be detailed with Gardasil (see Gardasil, The Vaccine).

The vaccine has been shown to have no therapeutic effect on the cervical lesions already present. However, what is not known is the effect the vaccine might have on the natural history of cervical lesions, in particular on the rate of recurrence or the clearance rate once treated.

The Cervarix efficacy data available have an average follow-up of five years, and antibody titers, which decline after the third dose but start plateauing after 18 months are still steady at five years. GSK believes that the AS04 adjuvant produces a stronger and more durable antibody immune response than amorphous aluminum hydroxyphosphate sulfate, the adjuvant used in Gardasil. It is currently conducting a study comparing Gardasil and Cervarix head-to-head. It is not possible for now to answer the question of duration of protection, and whether and when a booster will be needed.

7.3.3.3. Adverse Events

Table 7.9 summarizes the adverse events noted with Cervarix during the phase II study. Only local side effects were more common with Cervarix than with the adjuvant alone. This side-effect profile is not too dissimilar from that observed with Gardasil. In the PATRICIA trial, Cervarix had slightly more common general and local side effects than the HAV vaccine, 85.0% and 91.2%, respectively. The rates of unsolicited or adverse events, including chronic and autoimmune disorders were not different between the two groups. There was also no difference in the rate of premature births in the women in the two arms of the study who became pregnant.

7.3.4. Other Vaccines in Development

One anticipates the availability of more multivalent versions of the current L1 VLP vaccines. Such vaccines should have a much more drastic impact on reducing CIN, especially low grade CIN and ASC, than the current

Table 7.9 *Adverse Reactions with Cervarix*

	Cervarix (n = 531)	Adjuvant alone (n = 538)
Serious adverse events related to vaccine	0%	0%
Injection site reactions		
Pain[a]	94%	87%
Swelling[a]	34%	21%
Erythema[a]	36%	24%
Overall[a]	94%	88%
General symptoms		
Headache	62%	61%
Fatigue	58%	54%
Gastrointestinal	35%	32%
Pruritus	25%	20%
Rash	11%	10%
Elevated temperature	17%	14%
Overall	86%	85%
Withdrawal from study due to adverse events	0%	0.6%

[a]Statistically significant differences between the vaccine and placebo groups ($p < 0.001$).
Source: Data from Harper DM, Franco EL, Wheeler C, et al. Efficacy of a bivalent L1 virus-like particle vaccine in prevention of infection with human papillomavirus types 16 and 18 in young women: a randomized controlled trial. Lancet 2004; 364:1757–1765.

vaccines. If these vaccines are broadly deployed, then it is likely that cervical cancer screening will be profoundly affected. Vaccine cost will remain an issue, as these augmented vaccines are going to be more expensive to produce.

Cost being already a formidable barrier for the use of these VLP vaccines in the developing world, alternate vaccine options are being developed. One consists in expressing a slightly truncated version of the L1 polypeptide in *E. coli*, rather than in one of the more expensive eukaryotic expression systems, to produce imunogenic capsomeres and VLPs. A second approach relies on the fact that the N-terminus portion of the L2 polypeptide, which codes for the minor capsid protein, possesses neutralizing epitopes that appear to be broadly shared among all papillomavirus, and could thus provide a "universal" HPV vaccine. The problem to surmount is the poor immunogenicity of these polypeptides.

Table 7.10 Benefits of HPV Vaccination

- Reduced incidence of genital warts, CIN, cervical cancer
- Decreased morbidity from other HPV-related diseases
- Improved quality of life and survival
- Lower costs related to follow-up, diagnosis and treatment of cytological abnormalities
- Eventually less frequent HPV screening/testing intervals
- Reduced disparities in cervical cancer mortality if widespread vaccination is achieved

7.3.5. Benefits, Obstacles, and Strategies to Implement HPV Vaccination

7.3.5.1. Benefits (Table 7.10)

7.3.5.1.1. Decreased cervical cancer incidence The ultimate goal of the HPV vaccines is to reduce the incidence of invasive cervical cancer and other HPV-related diseases. A recent model by Kim and Goldie predicts that compared with the current practice of cervical cancer screening, routine vaccination of girls in the United States before the age of 12 years with a vaccine to prevent HPV types 6, 11, 16, and 18 would reduce the incidence of cervical cancer by 78% and reduce the rate of genital warts by 83%.

7.3.5.1.2. Cost-effectiveness Costs related to HPV disease stem from both the cost of treatment of cervical cancer and genital warts, but even more so, the costs related to screening and follow-up of low-grade cervical abnormalities. Studies in the United Kingdom, Australia, Mexico, the United States, Canada, and France, among others, have found that vaccinating 12-year-old girls with a quadrivalent HPV vaccine, combined with continued cervical cancer screening, is cost-effective in reducing the incidence of CIN, cervical cancer, and genital warts. Models corresponding to this scenario estimate vaccine costs at less than $50,000 per quality-adjusted life year gained (QALY), the cut-off that is generally accepted to make an intervention cost-effective, with one estimate as low as $3000. Countries with higher incidences of cervical cancer due to lower rates of screening derive the most per capita incremental benefit. Disparities in cervical cancer mortality could be reduced if widespread vaccination coverage is achieved. The duration of vaccine efficacy and whether a booster will be needed to provider life-long protection are the primary parameters that affect long-term costs. The cost-effectiveness of the vaccine decreases incrementally with older ages of women vaccinated. Initially, the greatest benefit is expected in the reduction of genital warts and CIN incidence, since cervical cancers take decades to develop. Adding the benefit of reducing non-cervical HPV-related conditions that is expected after vaccination with the quadrivalent HPV vaccine makes the cost-effectiveness ratios more favorable. One study estimates the cost of these conditions to be approximately $418 million in the United States. The majority of these costs relate to juvenile-onset recurrent respiratory papillomatosis, anogenital warts, and anal cancer.

7.3.5.1.3. Reduction in cytological screening Since neither HPV vaccine currently available covers all oncogenic HPV types, cytological screening for immunized individuals remains necessary. However, the frequency of screening can eventually be reduced or delayed until an older age (e.g., 24–25 years), once the cohort of vaccinated individuals ages into screening recommendations. As vaccination coverage improves, the incidence of precancerous lesions will decrease. Since the positive predictive value of testing will decrease, it will be more cost effective to reduce the recommended frequency of screening tests. This will also maintain a low rate of false positive cytological results.

7.3.5.2.Obstacles (Table 7.11)

7.3.5.2.1. Adolescent or parent

7.3.5.2.1.1. HPV knowledge While public knowledge about the causative effect of HPV on cervical cancer and genital warts has increased since approval of the HPV vaccine, many parents and adolescents remain unaware of these associations. Most also lack an understanding of the reasons to vaccinate prior to sexual activity.

7.3.5.2.1.2. Access to Care Throughout the world to varying degrees, access to healthcare is a barrier to adolescents' receipt of vaccines. Lack of knowledge of recommended vaccines, costs, time, and inconvenience associated with clinical visits, and concern about confidentiality are potential barriers to receipt of healthcare. In the United States adolescents have significantly fewer healthcare visits than younger children, and visits decrease with increasing age of adolescence until women reach child-bearing years. By then, most are sexually active and the vaccine is ineffective against HPV types to which the woman has already been exposed. A three-dose schedule presents a particular burden for a population with few visits.

7.3.5.2.1.3. Vaccine acceptability Studies performed in developing countries prior to the licensure of HPV vaccine showed that the majority of parents are willing to have their children vaccinated against HPV. Overall across studies, 6% to 12% of parents have mentioned a concern that HPV vaccine could promote adolescent sexual activity, and the media has highlighted this concern. Parent and adolescent opinions are most

Table 7.11 Obstacles to HPV Vaccination

Patient/parent or guardian	
HPV knowledge	• Unaware of HPV and cervical cancer association
	• Lack of understanding of reason for vaccinating at younger age
Access to care	• Infrequent healthcare visits
	• Cost, time, inconvenience, and confidentiality are barriers
Vaccine acceptability	• High rates of acceptability, few concerns about promoting sexual activity
	• Parents concerned with side effects, safety, efficacy, duration of effectiveness
Consent	• Parental consent generally required for vaccination
Provider Knowledge	• General practitioners and pediatricians have less HPV knowledge than obstetrician/gynecologists, and are the primary vaccinators
Vaccine acceptability	• High, but more willing to vaccinate older teens
Practice issues	• Time, compensation, consent all complicate delivery
Health Care System	
Cost/insurance coverage	• Expensive vaccine, private and public funding varies
	• Greater burden for developing countries
Infrastructure	• Lack of tracking systems, storage, cold chain, follow-up for doses 2 and 3

influenced by vaccine efficacy and safety, the recommendation of their physician, an understanding of their susceptibility to HPV disease and the severity of HPV infection and cervical cancer. For most parents, safety and trust issues are more important than socioeconomic background in measurements of vaccine acceptance. In developing countries, such as Mexico and Vietnam, parents support vaccination once they are educated about the link between HPV and cervical cancer, despite conservative attitudes toward premarital sex.

7.3.5.2.1.4. Consent   While adolescents are able to obtain other reproductive healthcare services without parental consent, in most countries, parental consent is required prior to vaccination. In the United Kingdom, one study estimated that if parental consent is mandatory for HPV vaccination, at least 20% of those under age 16 will not be vaccinated.

7.3.5.2.2. Healthcare provider

7.3.5.2.2.1. Knowledge Studies performed prior to licensure of the HPV vaccine showed that physicians demonstrated immense variability in their knowledge of HPV infections. Overall, general practitioners and pediatricians had less HPV knowledge than obstetrician/gynecologists.

7.3.5.2.2.2. Vaccine Acceptability While nurse practitioners, obstetrician/gynecologists, family practitioners and pediatricians endorse HPV vaccination, they were more willing to vaccinate older adolescents compared to younger teens, and girls more than boys.

7.3.5.2.2.3. Practice Issues Lack of time, a complicated agenda for adolescent care, lack of tracking systems for adolescent vaccination, missed opportunities for vaccination, insufficient compensation, and issues with consent contribute to lack of timely vaccination delivery.

7.3.5.2.3. Health care system

7.3.5.2.3.1. Cost/insurance coverage HPV vaccine is the most expensive recommended vaccine to date, at least €100 per dose for each of three vaccine doses. Given this, cost is a tremendous barrier to vaccine delivery. Funding for vaccination comes from both public and private sectors, but mechanisms vary by country. In the United States, the cost of HPV vaccination is primarily borne by private insurance companies and a federal program—the Vaccine for Children Fund—for children aged 18 and under who are uninsured or publicly insured. The cost of HPV vaccine is an even greater burden for developing countries where cervical cancer prevalence is much higher, due to lack of screening.

7.3.5.2.3.2. Infrastructure Lack of tracking systems in most countries for adolescent immunizations makes it difficult to recall patients who miss the initial vaccine or who are due for subsequent vaccine doses.

7.3.5.3. Strategies (Table 7.12)

7.3.5.3.1. Adolescent and parent

7.3.5.3.1.1. Education Broad-based HPV education is needed for the public to understand the link between HPV and cervical cancer. Education about the need for continued cytological screening (for the 25% of HPV types not covered by the vaccine) is necessary to maintain the low incidence of disease assumed in the studies mentioned above.

7.3.5.3.1.2. Access to care Universal vaccination is more likely to reach a majority of adolescents when delivered during early adolescence, when

Table 7.12 Strategies to Implement HPV Vaccination

Patient/parent or guardian	
Education	• Increase education (public media, health departments) to patients and parents about HPV and related diseases
	• Reinforce need for continued cervical cancer screening
Access to care	• Capitalize on high rates of school attendance for young adolescents
	• Encourage visits for adolescent preventive care
	• Consider mandating vaccine for school attendance in future
Vaccine acceptability	• Explain need, benefits, safety of vaccination
	• Emphasize role of cancer prevention
Consent	• Develop policies regarding vaccine consent
Provider Education	• Emphasize link between oncogenic HPV types and cancer of the cervix and other sites
	• Clear guidelines, educational programs from professional organizations, promote vaccine in early adolescence
	• Guidance to address parental concerns
	• Need for continued cervical cancer screening
Practice issues	• Avoid missed opportunities, use standing orders
Health Care System	
Cost/insurance coverage	• Ensure adequate reimbursement for vaccine providers
	• International programs to support neediest countries
Infrastructure	• Develop national immunization registries, reminder-recall systems for tracking
Access to care	• Provide adolescent-friendly clinics with confidential care

teens are more likely to access the healthcare system and their vaccination decisions are made for them by their parents. Schools may serve an important role in vaccinating a large number of adolescents since attendance rates are high for early adolescents, or in ensuring vaccination with school requirements, which are controversial.

7.3.5.3.2. Healthcare providers
7.3.5.3.2.1. Education   Strong recommendations from healthcare providers are known to be associated with increased vaccine uptake. Healthcare

providers look to their professional organizations for guidance, and educational programs and clear guidelines from these agencies likely has affected HPV knowledge and vaccine acceptance. These organizations can also provide guidance as to how to address potential parental concerns. Encouraging physicians to provide HPV vaccine in early adolescence by focusing on the individual and public health benefits of vaccination is important to provide the best protection possible from the vaccine.

7.3.5.3.3. Health care system

7.3.5.3.3.1. Cost/insurance   Public financing of the HPV vaccine is the best way to ensure that it will reach the targeted groups, as is occurring in Italy and Australia (Table 7.13) Ensuring that health insurance reimburses vaccination (as is occurring in Belgium, France, Germany, some U.S. states) also results in increased vaccination rates. Low-income countries may benefit from tiered pricing of the vaccine. Health officials from developing nations are discussing methods to obtain access to international financing mechanisms such as the Global Alliance for Vaccines and Immunizations (GAVI) to potentially subsidize the vaccine.

7.3.5.3.3.2. Infrastructure   Government support of infrastructure, including expanding the capacity for cold chain space (the uninterrupted chain of refrigerated storage spaces through which the vaccine moves from production to patient delivery), maintaining supplies and monitoring uptake is crucial to maintain a successful vaccination program. To ensure that the vaccine reaches the majority of the population, immunization information systems are necessary to track doses given. Major international organizations, including the World Health Organization, International AIDS Vaccine Initiative and the Program for Appropriate Technologies in Health (PATH) are analyzing methods of effectively delivering the HPV vaccine throughout the world.

7.3.6. Unanswered Questions

HPV vaccines have been introduced starting in 2006, their novelty leaves several questions unanswered. The following are among the most important.

7.3.6.1. HPV vaccination impact on cancer

The abundance and strength of the evidence establishing a causal link between HPV infection and cervical cancer is so strong that there is little doubt that cervical cancer will be reduced by HPV vaccination. Yet, this has to be documented. This will also provide the last remaining proof of a causal link. A phase IV study is already in place in the Nordic countries, but

Table 7.13 Sample of HPV Vaccine Recommendations and Funding, July 2008

Country	Vaccine recommendation	Funding
Australia	Girls in school aged 12–13, available to females to age 26	Universal free vaccination
Austria	Girls and women aged 9–26, and boys aged 9–15	Only one province offers the vaccine to females aged 9–26 at about half price through hospital clinics, other populations pay out of pocket
Belgium	Girls aged 10–13, catch-up of girls aged 14–26 if not sexually active	Partial funding through health insurance, reimbursement for catch-up aged 12–15
Canada	Age varies by province, 6th, 7th, or 8th grade girls	Publicly funded
France	Girls aged 14, catch-up for girls aged 15–23, before or within 1st year of sexual activity	Reimbursement by the National Security system at 65% cost of vaccination
Germany	Girls aged 12–17 before 1st sexual intercourse	Obligatorily reimbursed by health insurance
Ireland	Universal for 12-year-old girls	Universal free vaccination
Italy	Girls aged 12, catch up aged 25–26, may add cohort of 13–24	Free vaccination for all 12-year-olds Can pay a pharmacy with medical prescription if not covered by program
Netherlands	Girls aged 12, catch-up age 13–16	Publicly funded
Sweden	Girls aged 13–17	Reimbursed by insurance, co-payment by parents of <15%
United Kingdom	Girls aged 12–13, catch up to 18 years	Publicly funded
United States	Age 11–12 girls, catch-up age 13–26, can start as young as 9	Most private insurances Uninsured, public insurance: publicly funded to age 18

Source: Preparing for the introduction of HPV vaccine in the WHO European region: strategy paper. World Health Organization. http://www.euro.who.int/document/e91432.pdf (slightly modified).

one can be confident that other efforts will be made to address this question, particularly in geographic areas where cervical cancer has a high incidence. Nevertheless, because it takes approximately a couple of decades for cancer to develop from the time a high-risk oncogenic HPV infection is contracted, results are not expected for another decade. It will be important to also measure the impact of HPV vaccination on the other HPV-associated cancers of the anus, vulva, vagina, penis, and head and neck. Some are rare, and for that reason may be difficult to study, but some are rapidly increasing in incidence, especially anal and oropharyngeal cancers. They deserve close attention.

7.3.6.2. Vaccine effectiveness

Whereas the vaccine's efficacy is impressive and well demonstrated in women, its effectiveness—its impact on the health of the general population—needs to be better defined. It will depend on vaccine coverage, the proportion of girls and women that are seronegative and HPV DNA negative for the vaccine genotypes at vaccination, as well as on the exposure risk, which will evolve as herd immunity builds up. The greater the vaccine effectiveness, the greater the impact of vaccination will be on cervical cancer screening.

7.3.6.3. Breadth of HPV coverage

The current vaccines do provide protection against a key, but limited number of HPV genotypes, types 6, 11, 16, and 18 for Gardasil, and types 16 and 18 for Cervarix. The demonstration that they also confer a degree of cross-protection against two genotypes related to types 16 and 18, 31 and 45, respectively is a positive development. Altogether, these vaccines are already expected to be excellent preventive tools against HPV-associated cancers. However, 90% of the healthcare costs in the United States devoted to genital HPV diseases go to screening and follow-up of lesions that are not invasive cancers. Adding more genotypes to the HPV vaccine will be necessary to have the strongest impact on these costs.

7.3.6.4. Efficacy in men

The recent results of Gardasil in men have shown that it is very effective for the prevention of external genital warts, and possibly penile, perineal, and perianal intraepithelial neoplasias. Whether regulatory agencies will deliver an indication for males in unknown. In the US, it is not expected to occur before the fall of 2009. Once indicated for males, national advisory immunization committees will have to make recommendations on vaccine use, which in turn will determine reimbursement. The potential benefit of

HPV vaccination in males goes beyond genital warts, but also includes cancer of the anus, for which early studies are ongoing, cancer of the penis, and also cancer of the head and neck area, especially of the hypopharynx. The potential impact of male vaccination on these conditions will have to be taken into account in future cost-effectiveness assessments.

7.3.6.5. Efficacy and effectiveness in special populations

There is now evidence that Gardasil is effective in 27- to 45-year-old women. Data are needed in populations that are immunodeficient, especially those infected with HIV, or immunosuppressed, for example to prevent an allogeneic graft rejection or treat an autoimmune disorder. Recurrent respiratory papillomatosis is a rare but crippling disease, and it would be important to evaluate the impact on this disease of the HPV vaccination of young girls, and eventually young boys, but also of pregnant women with external genital warts or other genital HPV infections. The presence of antibodies in the birth canal, might be effective in reducing the rate of transmission of HPV during vaginal delivery.

7.3.6.6. Duration of efficacy

The actual duration of the protection given by the HPV vaccines is unknown, but is at least of five years. Already we know that a booster is very effective at inducing a rise in neutralizing antibodies that goes higher then the previous highest response. Nevertheless, avoiding a booster is highly desirable for this vaccine for reason of cost and delivery. The kinetics of anti-HPV VLP antibodies allows to expect a long durability. It will be of interest to try to ascertain whether natural infection will be a natural booster. If the vaccine HPV types progressively disappear, this putative natural booster might also disappear.

7.3.6.7. Impact of the HPV vaccine on HPV-associated disease natural history and HPV transmission

It is clear that the current HPV vaccines have no therapeutic effect on existing cervical lesions, and probably any other HPV-associated lesions. This is not to say that they do not impact on the recurrence or relapse rates of these lesions once treated, or prevent the development of new warts during standard treatment. These questions are pertinent, because recent reanalysis of the Gardasil Protocol 015 (FUTURE II trial) showed that the vaccine was 100% (95% CI: 29, 100) effective preventing CIN of all grades in subjects who were HPV DNA negative, but seropositive at entry. There was even a similar trend, with an efficacy of 22% (95% CI: 6, 42), in subjects who were HPV DNA positive and seronegative at entry.

7.3.6.8. HPV type replacement

Whether non-vaccine HPV types will replace those eliminated by vaccination is unanswered at the moment. However, there is no evidence so far that this has occurred in the vaccinated cohorts. What has been taken by some as a troublesome trend in the Gardasil trials was artifactual, and created by the way cases were counted (see Gardasil, phase III and IV studies, section 7.3.2.1.3.). HPV types coinfections are common, and do not appear independent events. In other words, the probability of having an infection by two different HPV types, is not the product of the probabilities of having an infection by either type alone. It is in fact higher, suggesting that there is a clustering effect. By eliminating the vaccine types, one would then expect to diminish the prevalence of the non-vaccine types that are associated with them. Even if type replacement does occur, it will be important to make sure that the phenomenon is not related to the ability of the HPV DNA tests (e.g., PCR) to better pick up in the absence of vaccine HPVs weak signals from non-vaccine HPV types.

7.3.6.9. Vaccine safety

So far the HPV vaccines appear to be very safe, with no serious illness or death that has been causally linked to vaccination. This vaccination is recent and there is a constitutive resistance to vaccination in people whose motivations range from a legitimate suspicion, informed by past episodes in the history of vaccines of unjustified dismissal of evidence, to plain irrationality and venality. Only time and continuing vigilance, in particular through post-marketing studies, will provide greater confidence in the vaccine's safety.

7.3.6.10. Vaccine accessibility

Gardasil and Cervarix are expensive vaccines, clearly an obstacle to their delivery to the developing countries where the incidence of some of the HPV-associated diseases, especially cervical cancer, is very high. This is not a new issue, and experience suggests that prices will eventually come down under the influence of various factors, including public pressure, the recovery of development costs, which are considerable, and possibly as cheaper alternate vaccines come to market. In the meantime, vaccine donations by the manufacturers (for example Merck has pledged in 2007 the donation of 3 million doses over the following 5 years to lower income countries), and subsidized vaccine distribution by the Bill and Melinda Gates Foundation have happened.

Selected References

Web Sites

Slides of the presentations made three times a year to the U.S. Advisory Committee on Immunization Practices (ACIP). They contain many current, otherwise unpublished information. Available at: http://www.cdc.gov/vaccines/recs/acip/slides.htm.

ACIP recommendations for the quadrivalent HPV vaccine (Gardasil). Available at: http://www.cdc.gov/mmwr/PDF/rr/rr5602.pdf.

Articles

Condoms

Bleeker MC, Berkhof J, Hogewoning CJ, et al. HPV type concordance in sexual couples determines the effect of condoms on regression of flat penile lesions. Br J Cancer 2005; 92:1388–1392.

Winer RL, Hughes JP, Feng Q, et al. Condom use and the risk of genital human papillomavirus infection in young women. N Engl J Med 2006; 354:2645–2654.

Gardasil General Review

Barr E, Sings HL. Prophylactic HPV vaccines: new interventions for cancer control. Vaccine 2008; 26:6244–6257.

Gardasil Phase I Studies

Brown DR, Fife KH, Wheeler CM, Koutsky LA, Lupinacci LM, Railkar R, et al. Early assessment of the efficacy of a human papillomavirus type 16 L1 virus-like particle vaccine. Vaccine 2004; 22:2936–2942.

Fife KH, Wheeler CM, Koutsky LA, Barr E, Brown DR, Schiff MA, et al. Dose-ranging studies of the safety and immunogenicity of human papillomavirus Type 11 and Type 16 virus-like particle candidate vaccines in young healthy women. Vaccine 2004; 22:2943–2952.

Poland GA, Jacobson RM, Koutsky LA, Tamms GM, Railkar R, Smith JF, et al. Immunogenicity and reactogenicity of a novel vaccine for human papillomavirus 16: a 2-year randomized controlled clinical trial. Mayo Clin Proc 2005; 80:601–610.

Villa LL, Ault KA, Giuliano AR, Costa RL, Petta CA, Andrade RP, et al. Immunologic responses following administration of a vaccine targeting human papillomavirus Types 6, 11, 16, and 18. Vaccine 2006; 24:5571–5583.

Gardasil Phase II Studies

Block SL, Nolan T, Sattler C, Barr E, Giacoletti KE, Marchant CD, et al. Comparison of the immunogenicity and reactogenicity of a prophylactic quadrivalent human papillomavirus (types 6, 11, 16, and 18) L1 virus-like particle vaccine in male and female adolescents and young adult women. Pediatrics 2006; 118: 2135–2145.

Koutsky LA, Ault KA, Wheeler CM, Brown DR, Barr E, Alvarez FB, et al. A controlled trial of a human papillomavirus type 16 vaccine. N Engl J Med 2002; 347: 1645–1651.

Olsson SE, Villa LL, Costa RL, Petta CA, Andrade RP, Malm C, et al. Induction of immune memory following administration of a prophylactic quadrivalent human papillomavirus (HPV) types 6/11/16/18 L1 virus-like particle (VLP) vaccine. Vaccine 2007; 25:4931–4939.

Reisinger KS, Block SL, Lazcano-Ponce E, Samakoses R, Esser MT, Erick J, et al. Safety and persistent immunogenicity of a quadrivalent human papillomavirus types 6, 11, 16, 18 L1 virus-like particle vaccine in preadolescents and adolescents: a randomized controlled trial. Pediatr Infect Dis J 2007; 26:201–209.

Villa LL, Costa RL, Petta CA, Andrade RP, Paavonen J, Iversen OE, et al. High sustained efficacy of a prophylactic quadrivalent human papillomavirus types 6/11/16/18 L1 virus-like particle vaccine through 5 years of follow-up. Br J Cancer 2006; 95:1459–1466.

Gardasil Phase III Studies

Ault KA. Effect of prophylactic human papillomavirus L1 virus-like-particle vaccine on risk of cervical intraepithelial neoplasia grade 2, grade 3, and adenocarcinoma in situ: a combined analysis of four randomised clinical trials. Lancet 2007; 369:1861–1868.

Garland SM, Hernandez-Avila M, Wheeler CM, Perez G, Harper DM, Leodolter S, et al. Quadrivalent vaccine against human papillomavirus to prevent anogenital diseases. N Engl J Med 2007; 356:1928–1943.

Joura EA, Leodolter S, Hernandez-Avila M, Wheeler CM, Perez G, Koutsky LA, et al. Efficacy of a quadrivalent prophylactic human papillomavirus (types 6, 11, 16, and 18) L1 virus-like-particle vaccine against high-grade vulval and vaginal lesions: a combined analysis of three randomised clinical trials. Lancet 2007; 369:1693–1702.

Koutsky LA. Quadrivalent vaccine against human papillomavirus to prevent high-grade cervical lesions. N Engl J Med 2007; 356:1915–1927.

Luna J, Saah A, Hood S, Bautista OM, Barr E, Investigators FI. Safety, efficacy, and immunogenicity of quadrivalent HPV vaccine (Gardasil) in women aged 24–45. Presented at: 24th International Papillomavirus Conference and Clinical Workshop, November 3–9, 2007; Beijing, China, 2007:PA1–04.

Siegrist CA, Lewis EM, Eskola J, et al. Human papilloma virus immunization in adolescent and young adults: a cohort study to illustrate what events might be mistaken for adverse reactions. Pediatr Infect Dis J 2007; 26:979–984.

Cervarix General Review

Keam SJ, Harper DM. Human papillomavirus types 16 and 18 vaccine (recombinant, AS04 adjuvanted, adsorbed) [Cervarix]. Drugs 2008; 68:359–372.

Cervarix Phase I Studies

Giannini SL, Hanon E, Moris P, Van Mechelen M, Morel S, Dessy F, et al. Enhanced humoral and memory B cellular immunity using HPV16/18 L1 VLP vaccine formulated with the MPL/aluminium salt combination (AS04) compared to aluminium salt only. Vaccine 2006; 24:5937–5949.

Cervarix Phase II Studies

Harper DM, Franco EL, Wheeler C, Ferris DG, Jenkins D, Schuind A, et al. Efficacy of a bivalent L1 virus-like particle vaccine in prevention of infection with human papillomavirus types 16 and 18 in young women: a randomised controlled trial. Lancet 2004; 364:1757–1765.

Harper DM, Franco EL, Wheeler CM, Moscicki AB, Romanowski B, Roteli-Martins CM, et al. Sustained efficacy up to 4.5 years of a bivalent L1 virus-like particle vaccine against human papillomavirus types 16 and 18: follow-up from a randomised control trial. Lancet 2006; 367:1247–1255.

Pedersen C, Petaja T, Strauss G, Rumke HC, Poder A, Richardus JH, et al. Immunization of early adolescent females with human papillomavirus type 16 and 18 L1 virus-like particle vaccine containing AS04 adjuvant. J Adolesc Health 2007; 40:564–571.

Cervarix Phase III Studies (see ACIP site)

Hildesheim A, Herrero R, Wacholder S, Rodriguez AC, Solomon D, Bratti MC, et al. Effect of human papillomavirus 16/18 L1 viruslike particle vaccine among young women with preexisting infection: a randomized trial. JAMA 2007; 298: 743–753.

Benefits, Obstacles, and Strategies to Implement HPV Vaccination

Brabin L, Greenberg DP, Hessel L, Hyer R, Ivanoff B, Van Damme P. Current issues in adolescent immunization. Vaccine 2008; 26(33):4120–4134.

Brewer NT, Fazekas KI. Predictors of HPV vaccine acceptability: a theory-informed, systematic review. Prev Med 2007; 45:107–114.

Kim JJ, Goldie SJ. Health and economic implications of HPV vaccination in the United States. N Engl J Med 2008; 359:821–832.

Zimet GD, Shew ML, Kahn JA. Appropriate use of cervical cancer vaccine. Annu Rev Med 2008; 59:223–236.

Index

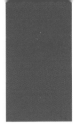